Beating the Flu

ALSO BY J.E. WILLIAMS

Viral Immunity
Prolonging Health
The Andean Codex

Beating the

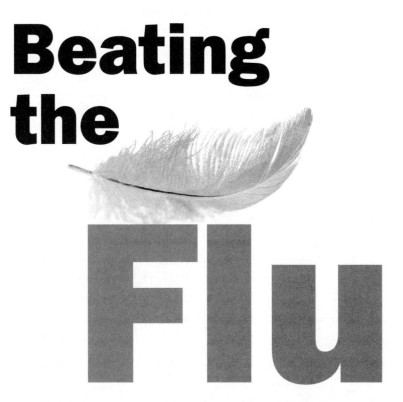

Flu

The Natural Prescription for Surviving Pandemic Influenza and Bird Flu

J.E. Williams, O.M.D.

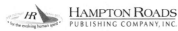

HAMPTON ROADS
PUBLISHING COMPANY, INC.

Cover design by Steve Amarillo
Cover digital imagery (c) Jupiterimages. All rights reserved.

Hampton Roads Publishing Company, Inc.
1125 Stoney Ridge Road
Charlottesville, VA 22902
434-296-2772
fax: 434-296-5096
e-mail: hrpc@hrpub.com
www.hrpub.com

If you are unable to order this book from your local
bookseller, you may order directly from the publisher.
Call 1-800-766-8009, toll-free.

Library of Congress Cataloging-in-Publication Data

Williams, J. E. (James Eugene), 1949-
  Beating the flu : the prescription for surviving pandemic influenza and
bird flu naturally / J.E. Williams.
       p. cm.
  Summary: "Dr. J. E. Williams examines the bird flu and offers advice
for avoiding it, as well as steps for overcoming the virus should you contract it. Dr. Williams argues that due to a shortage in antiviral pharmaceutical drugs, natural medicines will play a crucial role in minimizing
the outbreak"--Provided by publisher.
  Includes bibliographical references (p.   ).
  ISBN 1-57174-507-6 (5 1/2 x 8 1/2 tp : alk. paper)
  1. Avian influenza--Prevention. 2. Avian influenza--Treatment. 3.
Avian influenza--Alternative treatment. I. Title.
  RA644.I6W55 2006
  614.5'18--dc22
                                        2006016710

ISBN 1-57174-507-6

10 9 8 7 6 5 4 3 2 1

Printed on acid-free paper in the United States

DISCLAIMER

This book is written as a source of information to educate the reader. It is not intended to replace medical advice or care, whether provided by a primary care physician, specialist, or other healthcare professional including a licensed alternative medical practitioner. Please consult your doctor before beginning any new medications, diet, nutrients, or any form of health program. Dosages are given in ranges for the average adult and are to be used as guidelines only. Effects from any medications can vary widely from person to person, and applications must be adjusted to meet individual requirements.

The author has spent a great deal of time and energy supporting the information contained in this book with published documentation; however, this research is not intended to be used as justification for any of the recommendations contained in this book. The author has no financial ties to any of the products, clinics, services, or medications cited in the text or listed in the resource guide.

Neither the author nor the publisher shall be liable or responsible for any adverse effects arising from the use or application of any of the information contained herein, nor do they guarantee that everyone will benefit or be healed by these techniques or practices, nor are they responsible if individuals do not so benefit.

CONTENTS

Injectable Homeopathic Medicines • Injectable Chinese
Herbal Medicines • Blood Purification: The Hemopurifier

PREFACE

My intention in writing this book is to teach you how to beat the flu and survive pandemic influenza. I want you to take the bird flu situation seriously, but not panic. It's important to understand that your survival is not in the hands of fate, or governments, or multinational pharmaceutical companies. It's in your own hands. If you apply the simple, concrete, evidence-based natural solutions in this book in a timely manner, you will be prepared when the plague comes.

But before I discuss how to beat the flu, I'd like to tell you about me. For 35 years, I've espoused and practiced, in my research, clinical work, teaching, and personal pursuits, a way of life that proposes that biology and the practice of medicine be tempered with a reverence for nature and respect for intuition. Deep inquiry with an open, scientific mind and a true integrative medical approach is the answer to the questions confronting us as we draw the final battle line between disease and survival.

As a doctor of Oriental medicine, I've visited and studied in China and Hong Kong, the birthplace of influenza virus, since 1986. I know the profile of the virus and how it's treated by Western and traditional Chinese medicine. With more than 20 years of clinical experience, I learned its character and how the body responds to treatment. Because I recognized the seriousness of viral respiratory illness from my studies, travels, and clinical experience, more than a decade ago I started advising the public about the perils of an influenza pandemic. To teach people about viruses, I wrote an entire book, *Viral Immunity* (2002), about how to enhance your immune system to prevent and treat viral infections. To inform doctors so they are better able to help their patients, I published numerous papers and lectured at medical conferences on viral illnesses, viral immunity, and how to strengthen mucosal immunity against viral infection (the mucous membranes are the major viral entry portal).

The danger is real. No longer restricted to the exaggerated plots of bestselling novels and Hollywood movies, the possibility of a super flu pandemic is well within the realm of possibility.

The possibility is frightening. A pandemic super flu (an extremely deadly flu against which no one has natural immunity) could cover the globe in 250 days and conceivably infect 20 percent or more of the world's population of 6.6 billion. Extrapolating estimated deaths from 1918 mortality rates and factoring in human fatalities in Southeast Asia from bird flu in 2005, the death toll could reach an apocalyptic 360 million. Some say higher.

The problem is complicated and frightening. Influenza virus, one of our most ancient microbial adversaries, has evolved side by side with humans and, over the millennia, has learned to exploit weaknesses in our defenses to make us sick. It can outsmart our immune system, resist the drugs we've invented to kill it, and elude vaccines we employ to stimulate our immune systems to recognize it.

Avian influenza viruses are native to southern China, Hong Kong, and Southeast Asian countries, including Thailand and Vietnam. This humid tropical region where humans and domestic farm animals have lived in close proximity for thousands of years is the perfect incubator for microbes. Even ordinary flu starts among chickens and domestic waterfowl such as ducks and geese. It doesn't stay there, however. Influenza virus can jump to pigs and horses, and even people. Once in humans, it mutates rapidly into a pathogenic virus that spreads easily from person to person. Subsistence farmers will not easily change traditional farming practices and, until they do, megaviruses will continue to brew in China.

Conventional medicine and doctors are unprepared for a powerful and deadly flu pandemic. Until recently, doctors didn't treat commonly occurring viruses that cause a cold or the flu because the body's immune system neutralizes them better than drugs do. Ordinary flu, a nuisance disease to most of us, plays itself out in the body within a few weeks. A cold is over in about one week. Seasonal flu generally retains virulence for no more than several months during the average winter cold and flu season from November to April. By summer, it's gone.

Emerging influenza strains like H5N1 avian influenza, however, are not your ordinary flu. These new influenzas are highly contagious, cause horrific symptoms, and can kill within hours after infection.

To fight viral infections, the current biomedical paradigm uses expensive drugs and immunizations that are not effective, have potentially serious side effects, and are in short supply. The big pharmaceutical companies want us to believe that they're just a few years away from finding a cure. But can we trust the same companies that for decades have been promising a cure for cancer and an AIDS vaccine?

The solution is in our hands. Though influenza, in any of its many manifestations like the bird flu, can become a deadly human infection and there's no cure, there are ways to prevent and treat it using natural medicine. Natural medicines have a long history of successfully treating viral infections and there is now scientific evidence confirming their usefulness. Traditional Chinese medicine has been successfully treating influenza for thousands of years and in recent years has added scientifically proven antiviral herbal extracts to its medicine chest. European scientists have developed natural medicines manufactured to pharmaceutical standards. Herbs, vitamins and minerals, and natural biological compounds that activate the immune system's defenses can serve as part of an integrated prescription for beating pandemic influenza. In this way, you improve your chances of survival and those of your family and loved ones in the event of an influenza pandemic.

I care passionately about nature, the planet, global health, and the well-being of individual people. If I didn't, I wouldn't have spent decades and my own resources studying and practicing natural ways of health. My intention with this book is to share some of what I've learned and give you the power to beat the flu by putting true knowledge in your hands.

In the aftermath of a super flu pandemic, not only will individual people, perhaps even some of your family among them, require healing, but society and the entire world will need a time of recovery and introspection. It is my sincere hope that an influenza pandemic doesn't come soon, and when it does, that it's mild and not a super flu. Unfortunately, the likelihood that a pandemic will come is high. The bird flu has the potential to transform into a human flu and take pandemic form. If that happens, it is my wish that this book will have prepared you well.

To our survival and healing,
J. E. Williams, O.M.D., F.A.A.I.M.

INTRODUCTION

What You Will Learn in This Book

This book advises a sensible approach to immunization and antiviral drugs, and teaches you the best natural medicines to beat the flu. In it you will learn how to prevent infection and protect yourself and your family from the ravages of influenza.

Along the way in *Beating the Flu*, you will learn:

WHY THE EXPERTS AGREE THAT WE ARE IN FOR A FLU PANDEMIC AND POSSIBLY ONE OF EPIC PROPORTIONS.

WHERE INFLUENZA VIRUS ORIGINATES FROM AND WHAT TURNS A NUISANCE ILLNESS INTO A DEADLY DISEASE.

HOW VIRUSES MUTATE AND WHAT LESSONS WE'VE LEARNED FROM RECENT OUTBREAKS LIKE SARS AND PAST BIRD FLU PANDEMICS LIKE THE SPANISH FLU OF 1918.

WHAT BIRD FLU IS AND WHY IT'S SUCH AN OMINOUS DISEASE.

WHY VACCINES AND ANTIVIRAL DRUGS DON'T WORK AS WELL AS WE'RE LED TO BELIEVE, AND WHY THEY MIGHT NOT WORK AT ALL.

HOW TO STRENGTHEN YOUR BODY'S VIRAL IMMUNITY TO BEAT THE FLU.

WHICH FOODS ARE THE BEST FLU FIGHTERS.

WHAT ARE THE BEST IMMUNE-BOOSTING SUBSTANCES TO COUNTER THE FLU.

Beating the Flu

HOW TO USE THE MOST EFFECTIVE HERBAL, HOMEOPATHIC,
   AND OTHER NATURAL MEDICINES FOR BEATING THE FLU.
HOW TO OUTSMART THE FLU BY PERSONAL PREPAREDNESS.
WHY BIRD FLU SEEMS TO SELECT CHILDREN AND HOW TO
   PROTECT YOUR FAMILY FROM PANDEMIC INFLUENZA.
FIVE NATURAL PRESCRIPTIONS TO BEAT PANDEMIC
   INFLUENZA.

Part I explains the danger. You will learn what causes the flu and
the difference between ordinary flu and pandemic influenza. I discuss bird flu and why it could potentially become a human plague.
I also explain how to use antiviral drugs and vaccination wisely, but
caution that they may not work as well as pharmaceutical companies want us to believe they will.

Part II provides the solution. In this section of the book, I provide
detailed information on how to protect yourself and your family from
getting sick, what to do should you fall ill, and the best natural treatments. Drawing on my research and clinical experience, I provide
you with five natural-medicine prescriptions. I put the knowledge,
tools, and resources into your hands to help you beat the flu and survive a pandemic.

CHAPTER-BY-CHAPTER OVERVIEW

Chapter 1 explains the nature of pandemics, the seriousness of
the world's viral health situation, and what governments and public health agencies are doing to protect us from an influenza pandemic. Here, I discuss the potential of the appearance of a super flu,
an influenza pandemic so catastrophic that it's beyond the capacity
of scientists to conceive of and medical experts to deal with.

In chapter 2, you learn about influenza virus, why viruses are
becoming more lethal, and why antiviral drugs make them smarter.
The difference between cold and flu is explained so you can better
understand symptoms should you get sick. There's also an explana-
tion of the difference between ordinary flu and the symptoms of a
super flu.

Chapter 3 explains how influenza virus evolves and mutates into deadly strains. I discuss what a virus is, how they jump from animals to humans, and how a pandemic gets going. I also talk about the environmental dimension and ecological implications of an influenza pandemic.

Chapter 4 is specifically about avian influenza, H5N1 bird flu. I define what bird flu is and why it is the most likely virus to become a pandemic disease. In this chapter, I explain how sick you can get and just how fast a pandemic can spread globally and in your community.

In chapter 5, you learn who the main targets and carriers of influenza are, and how to steer clear of them so you don't get sick. Quarantine will only partially contain a fast-moving pandemic. I explain why it may not work at all, and why personal protection and knowledge of how to avoid infection may be your best bet.

Chapter 6 covers the benefits and weaknesses of immunization and antiviral drug therapy. I explain why it's unrealistic to rely exclusively on these high-tech solutions. Other medical options are presented that can help prevent dangerous secondary infections that can come with the flu.

Chapter 7 discusses the SARS (severe acute respiratory syndrome) outbreak and what we learned from the clash between modern hospital medicine and a new viral disease. I challenge Western drugs' effectiveness against viruses and review how the Chinese employed traditional herbal medicine and what we learned from using it on a large scale.

Chapter 8 teaches you how to strengthen your immune system to defend against the flu and learn the fastest way to strengthen your immune system against viruses. I explain how to use natural immune-boosting medicines such as colostrum and beta-glucan, as well as Chinese herbs such as astragalus.

In chapter 9, you learn about foods that boost your immunity and aid in treating flu symptoms. These include healthy soups and common kitchen spices, green tea, and garlic, as well as more exotic foods such as kimchi and umeboshi plums.

Chapter 10 outlines the most effective natural medicines to treat the flu. It discusses each medication in detail, informing you which ones provide optimal therapeutic benefit, what the most effective dosages are, and what the scientific evidence says about them. I explain the correct use of herbs such as echinacea and elderberry, homeopathic medicines such as Oscillococcinum, and anti-inflammatory herbs such as cat's claw. I cover Chinese herbs that beat the flu, including concentrated forms that are more potent than teas.

Chapter 11 provides detailed information about natural and biological medicines that require a licensed physician's skills to administer them. These medications take the treatment of serious infection to a level well beyond the scope of most books on natural therapies.

The last three chapters guide you through a step-by-step plan to prepare you for the event of a super flu pandemic. In chapter 12, I teach you how to prepare for a pandemic, what protective wear to use, and the best ways to treat the flu safely and effectively at home. In chapter 13, I discuss how to protect your family, especially children, from infection, how to care for those who do get sick, and how to care specifically for the elderly.

Chapter 14 guides you through a plan to prepare for the event of a super flu pandemic. I discuss the six most important aspects for a comprehensive strategy to beat the flu with natural medicines, and provide you with five prescriptions for survival.

ADDITIONAL MATERIAL TO HELP YOU BEAT THE FLU

At the back of the book, there is a glossary of terms; a list of informative websites, flu blogs, and other resources; and an extensive bibliography should you care to investigate the subject further.

AUTHOR'S NOTE ON CITATIONS

This book is based on 25 years of clinical experience, teaching, and up-to-date research. Though intended to educate and inform the reader, it was written primarily as a "how to" reference for prevention and treatment of influenza. To keep the text clear and simple, I've chosen to list the resources I used in the research for the book in a selected bibliography at the end, rather than interrupt the text with endless footnotes and citations.

PART I

THE DANGER
Pandemic Influenza
and Inadequate Protection

1
Phase Seven

The Makings of a Super Flu

Blue in the face, gasping for air, and fighting for life, the clinical picture of a super flu is not pretty. It starts like ordinary flu, the seasonal nuisance that causes fever, joint pains, malaise, and coughing. But this one is different. It progresses fast with a high fever and piercing headache. As your temperature rises, blood heats in the body core, muscles contract, and violent chills occur. You cannot get warm despite piles of blankets.

Once in the respiratory tract, the preferred ground for human influenza infections, the virus triggers a massive inflammatory reaction. Tissues die, blood vessels leak, and the lungs become filled with fluid. Coughing is violent and blood-tinged phlegm bubbles up into your throat and mouth. You gag and cough, and choke. In the end, viral pneumonia sets in; your lungs fail and you suffocate to death, choked by your own secretions.

WHAT'S A PANDEMIC?

The term *pandemic* refers to a global disease outbreak. In comparison, an *epidemic* is a fast-spreading disease that affects a group of people in a limited geographical area but doesn't affect global health.

A *flu pandemic* is a worldwide outbreak of a new strain of influenza virus that no one has immunity against and so it causes widespread sickness and loss of life. It's so contagious that the number of new cases increases exponentially.

The reason we don't have immunity to a newly emerging influenza strain is because our immune systems have not developed antibodies to that particular strain. Antibodies are special proteins that remember an infection's genetic signature or code and alert the immune system to mount a defense to fight the virus.

Technically, anti-influenza antibodies circulating in the blood recognize a specific protein, called a viral antigen, and chemically attach or bind to it. In the case of the flu, they bind to hemagglutinin, HA for short. It's called this because HA causes red blood cells, which contain hemoglobin (where the "hem" part of the term comes from), to clump together or agglutinate. HA plays the crucial role of helping the virus dock onto a host cell. By binding to HA, antibodies and other immune substances inhibit the virus from attaching to and infecting healthy cells.

But influenza is a smart virus. It continuously rearranges itself chemically and genetically so our immune system can't recognize it. Then the virus has full reign in virgin territory.

Eventually, our immune system mounts a defense, but only after the virus has made us sick. Sometimes the immune system goes too far. If it overreacts, which is often the case in younger healthy adults, a cytokine storm occurs in which the body's own disease-fighting chemicals set off a self-destructive cycle resulting in explosive tissue damage. In a matter of hours, you can be dead.

In a pandemic, death rates are high. In the twentieth century, there were three flu pandemics. Between 50 and 100 million people died of Spanish flu in 1918, two million from the 1957 Asian flu, and one million in 1968 from Hong Kong flu.

During the 1918 flu, 60 percent of the people of Nome, Alaska, died and some Eskimo villages were entirely wiped out. In Samoa, 20 percent of the population died, and many other South Pacific islands fared much worse. In some British boarding schools, up to 90 percent of children were sick and many died. Death rates were particularly high among pregnant women, with 70 percent succumbing to the illness. The highest rate of infection, however, was among the young and healthy. The disease spread particularly fast among enlisted men in the armed forces on both sides of the Atlantic during World War I.

Pandemics, like hurricanes, move faster than government aid workers or medical bureaucracies can respond. Though viruses are far less predictable than a hurricane, we have come to understand some of their patterns. With foresight, we might avoid the worst. That's the good news. The bad news is we'll get hit.

The flu season comes every year, as it has for thousands of years. That's ordinary flu. Epidemiologists, scientists who track diseases and study epidemics, agree that we are overdue for a viral pandemic of plague proportions. The most likely candidate is our old nemesis, influenza—nature's way of thinning the herd.

Experts believe that the current avian H5N1 influenza strain, "bird flu," has the potential to become a human pandemic in proportions that could dwarf the Spanish flu of 1918, which killed millions and is, to date, the deadliest influenza outbreak in modern history.

Flu hunters, influenza experts who follow viral outbreaks, identify hot spots, study the disease in the laboratory, investigate its genetic code, and create theoretical worst-case scenarios in order to understand the disease and predict its path, all agree on one thing: It's only a matter of time before the next outbreak happens. The question no one can answer is how severe it will be and when it will come. The experts hope that a pandemic influenza will be nothing more than a more severe version of seasonal nuisance flu, but they're not betting on it. Viral dynamics are a mystery. We could be in for a super flu.

Beating the Flu

During a pandemic, symptoms may not follow the usual course. If the coming one is anything like the 1918 influenza pandemic, inflammation may not be confined to the lungs, like regular flu, but could affect the brain, liver, and other body tissues. The virus could even bypass the respiratory system entirely. Entering the bloodstream, it could cause the liver and kidneys to fail, damage nerves, and rupture muscles. Many of the people who survive this flu may never fully recover. Signs that H5N1 is not like ordinary flu are already here. Infected with bird flu, one Vietnamese boy died in a coma, days after he was infected, with an inflamed brain but with clear lungs.

The World Health Organization (WHO) Global Influenza Preparedness Plan lays out six pandemic phases and recommendations for public health responses. In September 2005, WHO issued a Phase 3 warning declaring that a virus new to humans was causing infection, but had not yet reached a stage where it easily spread

PHASES OF PANDEMIC ALERT PERIODS		
ALERT PERIOD	**RISK TO HUMANS**	**PHASE NUMBER**
Inter-Pandemic Period	Low risk	PHASE 1
	Higher risk	PHASE 2
Pandemic Alert Period	Limited human cases	PHASE 3
	Increased human transmission	PHASE 4
	Significant human illness	PHASE 5
Pandemic Period	Efficient and sustained infection	PHASE 6

SOURCE: Current WHO Phase of Pandemic Alert, November 2005
http://www.who.int/csr/disease/avian_influenza/phase/en/

between people. It's the lowest rung of the pandemic alert ladder. Only a few months before, they thought we were at the tipping point, but flu officials pulled back from declaring Phase 4 (at which human-to-human transmission occurs) because, although they found clusters of human cases in Vietnam, they were unable to positively identify them as H5N1 influenza.

Meanwhile, bird flu had become endemic in large parts of Asia and it was making its way to Turkey. By March 2006, it exploded into Africa and Europe, infecting chickens, swans, and cats, but few humans. The flu hunters were close behind. They claimed that, though humans were becoming infected, the virus was still too inefficient to warrant escalating the alert. Phase 5 is marked by rapid spread of infection, and the last rung, Phase 6, is when it goes global. There is no Phase 7; beyond Phase 6 is apocalyptic.

THE INFECTION OF THE WORLD

Viruses respect no boundaries. They recognize no international borders or time zones. They have no obligation to country, race, social status, gender, or age. Rich and poor alike become victims. They infect the young and the old. If given the opportunity, viruses travel long distances, circling the globe in days. They are everywhere and infect everything from bacteria to whales, and kill plants as well as people. No one has bulletproof immunity.

For a flu pandemic to occur, at least three concurrent if not simultaneous events are necessary: (1) a new highly aggressive virus has to appear with the ability to infect humans; (2) a vulnerable population must be available without previous exposure and no immunity to the new virus; and (3) infection has to spread readily and rapidly from person to person.

If a pandemic influenza strain like a human version of bird flu were to emerge, experts agree that global spread is inevitable. What makes this virus particularly ominous is that it travels on the wings of migratory birds and can be transported to market in live chickens and ducks. Once infected, people could carry it to other countries in a matter of hours when flying by airplane or traveling by bus or train.

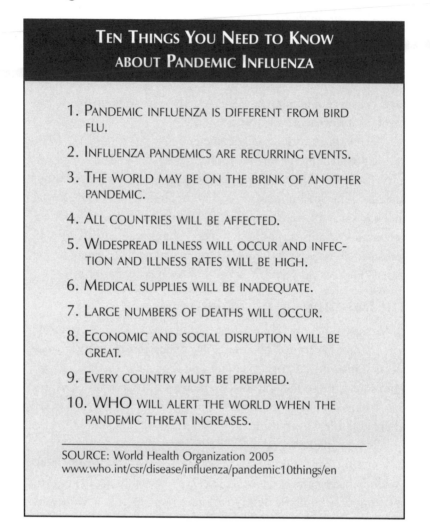

TEN THINGS YOU NEED TO KNOW ABOUT PANDEMIC INFLUENZA

1. PANDEMIC INFLUENZA IS DIFFERENT FROM BIRD FLU.

2. INFLUENZA PANDEMICS ARE RECURRING EVENTS.

3. THE WORLD MAY BE ON THE BRINK OF ANOTHER PANDEMIC.

4. ALL COUNTRIES WILL BE AFFECTED.

5. WIDESPREAD ILLNESS WILL OCCUR AND INFECTION AND ILLNESS RATES WILL BE HIGH.

6. MEDICAL SUPPLIES WILL BE INADEQUATE.

7. LARGE NUMBERS OF DEATHS WILL OCCUR.

8. ECONOMIC AND SOCIAL DISRUPTION WILL BE GREAT.

9. EVERY COUNTRY MUST BE PREPARED.

10. WHO WILL ALERT THE WORLD WHEN THE PANDEMIC THREAT INCREASES.

SOURCE: World Health Organization 2005
www.who.int/csr/disease/influenza/pandemic10things/en

Pandemic flu tends to spread in two or three waves in the course of a year. The first wave introduces the virus into a host population. Some people get violently sick and many die. The second wave, which follows three to nine months later, tends to be more deadly than the first or third, and many people get sick and die. By the third wave, our immune systems have developed specific antibodies and faster recognition occurs. It can defeat the virus before it invades too deeply in our tissues, and thus the virus is not as deadly. By the end of a year to a year and a half, it's over.

Medical scientists are as certain as they can be that, at some time in the future, we will experience another pandemic. It could be this year, next year, or in ten years. We don't know when it will come, but it is imminent.

Early detection and control are important to contain contagion and slow down the spread of infection. That may be only possible in the developed world where sufficient infrastructure, staff, equipment, communications, and medicines to cope with large numbers of sick people are available. Smaller countries like Switzerland are better off in this regard. The United States, though the richest country in the world, is a large country with pockets of high density where people live in Third World conditions, making inner cities and poor rural areas likely to be hit hardest. What transpired in New Orleans after Hurricane Katrina was an example of the poorest being most victimized. Lesser developed nations are even more vulnerable because of overcrowding, unsanitary personal hygiene, lack of medical services, and inadequate public health measures.

Of the three components necessary for a pandemic, the first two are nearly in place. H5N1 bird flu is a lethal virus that has the ability to become a human infection to which no one has immunity. To make matters worse, many social and economic conditions are in place for an epic disaster. Poverty and malnutrition caused by poor diet weaken immunity, and massive overcrowding in Third World slums makes for a perfect target. Widespread infection is certain to occur.

WHAT MAKES A SUPER FLU?

Infection from influenza virus is simple, effective, and universal. If you breathe, you can catch it. If a strain of influenza emerged that retained these traits and added others like resistance to antiviral drugs and the ability to outsmart vaccines, we'd be in big trouble.

A super flu is a viral infection that has all the ancestral traits of influenza, is drug-resistant, has undergone genetic mutations that make it possible for it to spread from human to human, no one has immunity to, and is extremely contagious and virulent. Pandemic influenza, like the Spanish flu of 1918, is much more virulent than regular flu. As if it is in a hurry to bypass the usual incubation period, it spreads readily and rapidly from person to person, and the infected individual can die within 48 hours after primary infection.

DIFFERENCES BETWEEN ORDINARY FLU AND PANDEMIC FLU	
ORDINARY	**PANDEMIC**
Body has viral immunity	No one is immune
Body not overwhelmed by virus	High viral load— body overwhelmed
Contagious	Highly contagious with easy transmission
Rare complications	Readily and rapidly progresses to pneumonia
Rarely fatal (less than 2%)	Can be fatal (possibly more than 50%)
Virus confined to respiratory tract	Can infect brain and other organs

When recreated in the laboratory, the 1918 flu virus was found to be 50 times more prolific than ordinary flu on the first day of infection, and 39,000 times more virus particles were released four days later. This is an astounding rate of replication and beyond what even the strongest of human immune systems can keep up with. It's no wonder that all of the mice used in the experiment died within six days. This is a forewarning of what a super flu pandemic would be like in humans. Almost no one infected would survive.

Were a super flu to attack, it is conceivable that more than half the population of India and regions of China and Southeast Asia would get sick. Japan, being an island and having the wealth to pour into medical resources, would fare better. Much of the Caribbean, Mexico, and many parts of Latin America would be infected. Countries like Haiti would be devastated. Africa, already suffering from AIDS and malaria, could receive a deathblow overshadowing famine and genocide. Western Europe, geographically close to Africa and contiguous to Russia, which in turn borders Asia, could be hit very hard. Many European countries, however, are preparing for the worst by stockpiling supplies of antiviral and other drugs to treat flu and secondary infections.

North America will not be spared. American bureaucracy will slow relief efforts, and politicians, unfamiliar with public health crisis, will be powerless. Centralization of resources will prevent rapid distribution of food and medicines. Natural disasters have been low on federal priorities. Hurricane Katrina showed us that nature is more powerful than terrorists and more unpredictable, even if we know the trajectory.

A tear in the fabric of society is upon us. With the breakdown brought about by a super flu, borders would be closed and international flights suspended. Schools and other places where people come in close contact, like theatres, would also be closed. National security may become vulnerable; insurgency and terrorism might escalate. Entire cities may need to be quarantined. The estimated costs of a flu pandemic in the United States alone are 70 to 165 billion dollars. The global economy, so much a part of the twenty-first century, would shut down.

In fact, super viral diseases are historically real. During the conquest of the Americas, upward of 95 percent of indigenous people in North America, Mexico, the Caribbean, Central America, and South America were wiped out by smallpox and influenza. The last major killer pandemic, the Spanish flu of 1918, caused an estimated 50 million deaths and possibly as high as 100 million in a single year. It reached even remote corners of the globe.

The 1918 Spanish flu pandemic was more like a Biblical

prophecy come true than a medical disease. Almost a century later, epidemiologists still study this worst of modern influenza pandemics for clues to help them understand and prepare for the next big one. What they have found has them scared: The 1918 flu was a type of bird flu.

Among domestic poultry and some wild migratory waterfowl, bird flu is devastating. It kills almost all birds infected and it's spreading around the world at an alarming rate. Of humans who have contracted the bird flu directly from handling sick chickens or ducks, half have died. It's no wonder flu experts are concerned.

A human flu pandemic would be as devastating but on a global scale. Contagion would be spontaneous. Infection would be swift and deadly. More than half of its victims would die painfully. In pandemics, an estimated 25 percent of the work force is unable to work. During a super flu pandemic, 30 to 50 percent of the population could become ill with influenza. World leaders, generals, and heads of corporations would become sick, just as would ordinary people including firefighters, police, and healthcare workers. The economies of some countries would be shattered.

Schools would close. Public transportation would grind to a halt. Store shelves would be empty and not be restocked for weeks. Martial law could be needed to control rioting and looting. Local police would not have adequate manpower to maintain law and order. Troops might be used to enforce quarantines and curfews.

Wall-to-wall cases would swamp hospital emergency rooms. To prevent overcrowding, triage hotlines may be used to sort the most serious cases from the merely sick and disabled. MASH-type field units would be set up in hospital and shopping mall parking lots and temporary influenza hospitals would have to be created in public buildings when hospitals overflow with patients. Many people would receive no formal medical care and would suffer and die in their homes. It's conceivable that entire families could die without anyone knowing. Rescue workers would have to go house to house, recovering bodies.

In some cities in poor states and in many small poor countries, the number of sick and dying people could reach catastrophic levels, totally outstripping city and governmental resources. Disposing of the dead would become a nightmare.

ARE WE PREPARED?

The prospect of catastrophic sickness is frightening. The scale of damage that nature can inflict is beyond what policy makers care to imagine. There are many questions, but few clear answers. How can a nuisance illness rise to plague proportions? When it arrives, will we be prepared? WHO experts inform us that we are not well prepared.

The United States has no wide clinical use of rapid in-office testing for flu as do the Japanese. We don't have enough antiviral drugs as does Hong Kong. We're not as organized as the Swiss. Even if we had sufficient antiviral drugs, they don't work that well and if improperly or overused could trigger a super flu mutant strain worse than the original one. There won't be enough vaccine to go around. Even if we make a safe and effective vaccine in time, it won't completely halt the spread of infection. There are not enough respirators and other medical supplies to assist the breathing of the most seriously ill.

American doctors aren't prepared. They have little training and almost no experience with severe infectious disease. They rely on symptom discrimination to diagnose and treat disease rather than cutting it off at the root. Many don't bother differentiating between a cold and the flu. Most consider the flu a self-limiting, nuisance illness that has no cure. Seasonal upper respiratory cases are so common that professional apathy is high. Antibiotics are indiscriminately prescribed. But antibiotics, designed to kill bacteria, don't touch viruses.

A pandemic tends to kill people at the extremes of the life span and persons with underlying chronic disease. In the elderly, who have the highest mortality rate from seasonal influenza, secondary infections like pneumonia are treated with antibiotics and lung inflammation with steroids. Comfort measures like oxygen are given to ease congestion and help breathing, and ventilators are used to assist failing lungs, but the elderly die anyway. Nursing homes, where aged people are warehoused, are particularly vulnerable, as are the healthcare workers who tend to our frail seniors. During a super flu pandemic, we could lose up to 90 percent of our elders.

If we are not prepared now, will we learn so we are ready the next time? Pandemics behave as unpredictably as the viruses that cause them. In previous pandemics, great variations were seen in mortality, severity of illness, and patterns of spread. During a pandemic, there is a huge surge in the number of cases, with an exponential increase over a very brief time, often in a matter of weeks. A pandemic strain's capacity to cause severe disease in traditionally unaffected age groups, namely, young adults, is a major determinant of a pandemic's overall impact. For example, firefighters and nurses tend to be younger, and if they become sick, emergency response is compromised.

In the best-case scenario, we'll see it coming, identify it early, and slow it down at the source. Asia is the most likely starting place, but it could happen anywhere or even in multiple places simultaneously. If we are lucky, the flu strain will be vulnerable to existing antiviral drugs and there will be enough supply. If we are lucky, we'll get the vaccine right the first time and there will be enough shots at the right dosage to inoculate key people and the most vulnerable groups, reducing the overall death rate. I'm sorry to say that this is overly optimistic and perhaps fantasy thinking.

Given time, an influenza virus will outsmart antiviral drugs. Many have done so already. When a virus becomes impervious to drugs, no one is immune. It may mutate so fast, scientists aren't able to keep up. A super flu could spawn multiple variant strains appearing simultaneously in different parts of the world. A super flu pandemic will not only kill animals and individual humans, but infect modern civilization. It will stop only when our immune systems learn to normalize it.

Your best bet to beat pandemic influenza is to educate yourself, develop a personal preparedness plan, protect your family, use prescription and over-the-counter drugs wisely, and learn to beat the flu naturally when it comes.

2
The Perfect Plague

Why Influenza May Be Nature's Most Successful Virus

Old foes don't die easily. In the case of influenza, it comes every year just like hurricane season. And like hurricanes, every century or so it attacks with a vengeance. Typically, influenza is a commonly occurring cold-weather nuisance disease that causes self-limiting respiratory infections. Fortunately, it doesn't come at the same time as hurricanes, which are summer storms.

Seasonal flu lasts from November to April and every year in the United States flu infects between 5 and 20 percent of the population, sends 200,000 to the hospital, kills about 36,000 people, and costs 15 billion dollars. Most fatal cases involve the elderly, infants and young children, and those weakened from stress and other diseases, especially chronic respiratory conditions like asthma and emphysema. Those older than 65 are particularly vulnerable and 90 percent of flu-caused deaths occur in individuals from this age group.

Influenza is such a successful virus that each year almost everyone on Earth is exposed, and about a third of us catch it. But it's by no means harmless. Worldwide, it kills between 50 and 200 people per million every year.

Flu can kill in several ways. It can destroy your lungs or damage them so much that bacteria overwhelm them with infection and you suffocate to death. Another way it kills is when your immune response to the virus triggers an inflammatory crisis that spirals out of control, destroying vital tissue in your heart, liver, kidneys, or brain.

WHAT'S INFLUENZA?

Influenza is a disease caused by a virus with an affinity for the nose, sinus passages, throat, and lungs of humans. Other animals get the flu. Pigs, horses, tigers, seals, and birds also catch it. Once in the respiratory tract, the virus multiples in the epithelial cells lining the mucous membranes, destroying the tiny hairs that help clean the airway passages.

Then individual influenza viruses, called virons, burrow into the tissue with the goal of finding a vulnerable cell. A single influenza viron is spherical in shape and covered by several hundred symmetrical protein spikes. These projectiles play a role in the way a single viron docks on and then enters a living cell. After docking on a live cell, a sequence of biochemical events takes place that ends with the genetic material of the virus being transported into the nucleus of the host cell. Here, the virus reassembles itself, replicates, and spreads to other cells. What makes us sick is the result of millions of influenza virons fighting it out with immune cells and chemicals in our body.

WHAT CAUSES THE FLU?

"True" flu, or influenza, is caused by an RNA virus from the *Orthomyxoviridae* family. *Myxo* is derived from the Greek for mucus; *ortho* means "true." The illness caused by this virus family is distinct from others that cause similar symptoms, as in the common cold or bronchitis.

There are three main types of influenza viruses: A and B belong to one group, and the C type, which rarely infects humans, belongs to another. There are also other strains that don't infect people. Influenza A virus is the most important as a human disease and has many subtypes.

The technical designation for influenza viruses uses a system of letters and numbers based on the formation of the two different protein spikes that occur on the external surface of the virus particle, or viron. Hemagglutinin spikes are designated H and neuraminidase spikes as N. Since 1980, a sequential numbering system has been employed: H1–H16 and N1–N9. Only five types of influenza are known to infect humans: H1, H2, H3, and N1 or N2. The avian influenza viruses H4, H5, and H7 make birds sick but usually don't infect humans. That may be about to change, however.

In addition to its technical designation, when the flu becomes a human infection, each of the different influenza A viruses is given a common name corresponding to the place of outbreak or origin: the Spanish flu of 1918 or the Hong Kong flu of 1968.

The word "influenza" is derived from the Latin *influentia*, to influence. During the Renaissance, astrologers in Florence attributed epidemic respiratory infections to the influence the stars had on people. Traditionally, seasonal flu is associated with an attack of cold weather. In Spanish, the seasonal flu is called *la grippe*. In China, it is called *ganmao*, whereas severe febrile diseases like SARS and pandemic influenza are termed *wen bing*.

SYMPTOMS OF THE FLU

A disease causes symptoms. In the case of influenza, there are no symptoms immediately after infection. With little warning, two to three days later, chills and shivering, malaise, aching, coughing, and headache begin. The body responds. Specialized immune cells spring into action producing chemical substances called cytokines (e.g., interleukin-6 and interferon).

Beating the Flu

The initial response of the immune system is intense, at times more violent than the infection itself. Fever, headache, cough, and body aches are the typical symptoms caused by the flood of immune chemicals. The throat and upper airways, the preferred places of entry, become inflamed, swollen, and sore.

Once in the respiratory passages, the virus replicates rapidly, and myriad cells become infected. They rupture and countless dying cells spill toxic residues into the bloodstream. The lymphatic system becomes flooded and lymph nodes in the neck and throat swell and become tender. As more immune chemicals and cells respond, fatigue and listlessness set in. You become sick and wish to remain in bed.

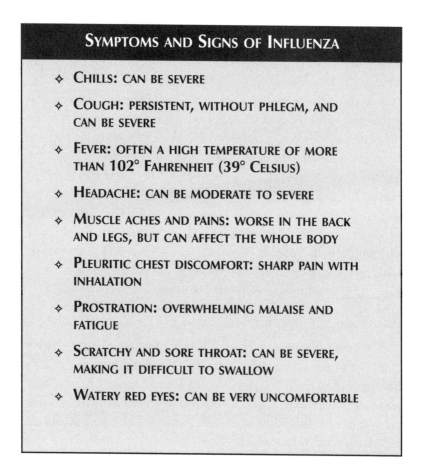

SYMPTOMS AND SIGNS OF INFLUENZA

✦ CHILLS: CAN BE SEVERE

✦ COUGH: PERSISTENT, WITHOUT PHLEGM, AND CAN BE SEVERE

✦ FEVER: OFTEN A HIGH TEMPERATURE OF MORE THAN 102° FAHRENHEIT (39° CELSIUS)

✦ HEADACHE: CAN BE MODERATE TO SEVERE

✦ MUSCLE ACHES AND PAINS: WORSE IN THE BACK AND LEGS, BUT CAN AFFECT THE WHOLE BODY

✦ PLEURITIC CHEST DISCOMFORT: SHARP PAIN WITH INHALATION

✦ PROSTRATION: OVERWHELMING MALAISE AND FATIGUE

✦ SCRATCHY AND SORE THROAT: CAN BE SEVERE, MAKING IT DIFFICULT TO SWALLOW

✦ WATERY RED EYES: CAN BE VERY UNCOMFORTABLE

Coughing due to bronchial irritation can last several weeks after the acute infection is over. Occasionally, a lingering cough and fatigue last as long as a month after infection. Rarely, nerve and muscle damage occurs.

When influenza invades the lungs, it can cause viral pneumonia. In susceptible people, bacteria, especially *Staphylococcus* species, cause secondary infection that can lead to death within two to three days due to tissue breakdown, accumulation of mucus and fluid, difficulty breathing, and lack of oxygen.

In routine infection, without pneumonia and its consequences, specialized white blood cells (cytotoxic T-cells and macrophages) clean up the airways after the body beats back the virus and play an important role in recovery.

Severity of symptoms depends on the type and virulence of the virus and the age, health status, stress level, and immunity of the person. Depending on how these factors play out during infection, the flu may pass with hardly any symptoms, make you sick enough so you can't work for several days, or kill.

IS IT A COLD OR THE FLU?

It's not always easy, even for a doctor, to distinguish between a cold and flu. In fact, the difference between the two is not covered in detail in medical textbooks for doctors in training and there are many misconceptions. Let's discuss the differences and clear up some of the misconceptions. It's important to distinguish between the two because treatment options, especially during a pandemic when medicines may be in short supply, are specific for each.

The common cold is caused by rhinoviruses (*rhino* means "nose"), which are distinctively different from those that cause the flu. The common cold and flu share the status, however, of being the most universal cause of respiratory tract infections in humans. In fact, approximately one-third of all complaints seen by doctors are for upper respiratory tract infections. On average, an adult will have two to five colds a year. If you're healthy and young, you might not get sick for several years. Stress weakens the immune system, making you more vulnerable to catching a cold or the flu. The aging process makes one more vulnerable because immunity weakens as you age.

After an incubation period of two to three days, typical cold symptoms begin. They start in the head with headache, pain and stiffness in the back of the neck, nasal congestion, sneezing, and sometimes chills and sore throat with the discharge of phlegm. Rarely is there fever. A cold peaks in a few days and is gone in a week.

Flu, on the other hand, comes on strong. It starts with a fever, headache, scratchy and sore throat, loss of appetite, and whole body aches; progresses to dry coughing; and is accompanied by malaise and weakness.

Both a cold and the flu can start with a scratchy throat. When you have the flu, a sore throat can be severe. A cold is mostly associated with headache and nasal congestion, however, whereas the flu is associated with coughing because the virus attacks the lungs. Therefore, the best clinical predictors of the flu are fever and cough, and severe sore throat.

Bacteria infections often follow behind the flu like buzzards circling a kill. These germs can cause sinus infections, tonsillitis, and pneumonia. There are few complications of a cold. Doctors are taught that dark yellow or green phlegm indicates bacterial infection, whereas clear, white, or light yellow phlegm is associated with viral infection. There is, however, no scientific evidence to support this notion. In fact, the yellow and green phlegm comes from the color of dead white cells and may reflect severity of inflammatory airway disease, not bacterial infection. High fever is associated with infection. If a fever is present along with dark-colored phlegm, a bacterial infection may be festering and antibiotics or antimicrobial herbs are clinically indicated. If there is no fever, rather than using antibiotics, as is the standard clinical practice, an anti-inflammatory medication or natural therapies may work better.

HOW IS THE FLU DIAGNOSED?

Typically, the diagnosis of flu is based on the clinical presentation. Because colds and the flu share common symptoms, and some bacterial infections produce similar symptoms, your doctor calls all

	COLD VERSUS FLU	
SYMPTOMS	**COLD**	**FLU**
Aches & Pains	Mild	Common and can be severe
Chest Congestion	Mild to moderate	Common and severe
Chills	Mild or absent	Common and can be severe
Cough	Hacking	Common and can be severe
Exhaustion	Never	Early and can be severe
Fever	Rare	High (101° F and higher)
Headache	Rare	Prominent
Sneezing	Typical	Sometimes
Sore throat	Common	Sometimes
Stuffy nose	Common	Sometimes, but can be severe
Weakness	Mild and short-lived	Common; lasting 2-3 weeks

flu-like viral illnesses acute upper respiratory tract infections (URIs). The appearance of many cases in a localized area during the winter when a known influenza virus is circulating among the population is strongly suggestive that the patient has the flu.

Rapid laboratory tests that use a throat swab are valuable in diagnosing dangerous influenza outbreaks and have become essential in the post-SARS (severe acute respiratory syndrome) world of emerging infections. These tests can confirm a diagnosis of influenza A in 30 minutes, though they can't differentiate what subtype it is. Until recently, these tests were rarely used in the average medical clinic or hospital. One problem yet to be overcome is that they are not always accurate. Missing the mark may be acceptable with ordinary flu, but it could cost lives during a pandemic.

Fast and accurate testing for specific influenza types could make a difference during a flu pandemic when medications are in short supply. Rapid identification could target cases most likely to bene-fit from antiviral drugs. There are, however, very few WHO-approved reference laboratories in the United States that are capable of making a diagnosis for influenza A, subtype H5 viruses—the type that causes bird flu.

In addition, there are few clinical studies comparing flu symp-toms to laboratory testing for influenza. Doctors agree that clinical findings identify patients with flu-like respiratory illness but are not particularly useful for confirming or excluding a specific diagnosis of influenza. These diagnostic discrepancies are not that important for ordinary flu, but during an outbreak become critical. To be pre-pared, clinicians should keep current with information from WHO and the U.S. Centers for Disease Control and Prevention (CDC) to find out if influenza is circulating in their communities. Prepared with this information, they are better able to treat patients with influenza-like illness empirically or to obtain a rapid influenza test that will assist with medical management decisions.

What's the Conventional Medical Treatment for Flu?

There's no cure for influenza. Though for some the flu can be fatal, ordinary seasonal flu is not a serious illness for the average healthy adult. Since few are worse for the experience (it may even help strengthen our immunity), doctors consider it a nuisance ill-ness. Conventional allopathic medicine has no good remedy for the flu. Treatment, therefore, is aimed at managing symptoms, rather than addressing the cause. Over-the-counter remedies are generally prescribed to make the patient as comfortable as possible until the flu passes, which it does in a week or two.

Rest and fluids help the body fight the virus and recover.

Acetaminophen lowers fever. For aches and pains associated with the flu, doctors recommend nonsteroidal anti-inflammatory medications such as aspirin and ibuprofen. These drugs help take away headache so you can sleep. Children between 6 and 12 years old should not take aspirin for flu symptoms because they can develop Reye's syndrome, a rare condition that targets the brain and liver, causing confusion, seizures, coma, or even death.

Respiratory symptoms can be managed with a variety of over-the-counter medications: decongestants so you can breathe better, expectorants to loosen up chest congestion, and antihistamines to dry up running secretions from your eyes and nose. If you're coughing a lot, a cough suppressant with dextromethorphan is prescribed to help quell the hacking. When coughing is severe, your doctor may prescribe a cough suppressant with codeine. Cough drops and throat lozenges help soothe mildly sore and tickly throats. If you are having trouble breathing due to severe lung inflammation, your doctor may prescribe a steroid drug.

Antiviral drugs are not commonly used for several reasons. First, only four antiviral drugs are approved by the U.S. Food and Drug Administration (FDA) for the treatment of influenza. Second, they don't work that well. To be effective at all, they have to be taken within the first 48 hours after symptoms start. Even then, they don't cure the flu but only reduce symptoms and shorten the duration of sickness by one or two days. Most people don't come in for treatment until their symptoms are severe, however, and that's usually past the window of therapeutic opportunity. Third, antiviral drugs have side effects.

Two of these antiviral drugs, amantadine and rimantadine, can cause nervousness, anxiety, insomnia, and light-headedness, as well as more severe adverse effects such as seizures and delirium. Some people experience nausea and lack of appetite. Because of these side effects, most doctors in years past were reluctant to use these drugs. In addition, influenza viruses have learned how to skirt their actions. Because disease resistance has become common, the CDC advises doctors not to use amantadine and rimantadine for prevention of the flu or against bird flu.

The other two antiviral drugs, zanamivir and oseltamivir phosphate, also have side effects. Zanamivir is rarely used because taking it is inconvenient. It is a powder that has to be inhaled utilizing a special device. It can cause allergic reactions including facial swelling and difficulty breathing, and is not recommended for people with asthma. Oseltamivir phosphate (Tamiflu) is the number one doctor recommended flu drug. It is a relatively new drug, however, and hasn't been tested extensively. Also, some influenza viral strains are already resistant to its effects. Side effects include severe skin reactions, nausea, vomiting, and dizziness. None of these drugs has been shown to be safe for pregnant women, unborn fetuses, or during nursing.

WHAT ARE THE COMPLICATIONS OF THE FLU?

Because influenza is caused by a virus, antibiotics don't kill it. Antibiotics treat bacterial infections such as bronchitis and pneumonia. Many different types of bacteria can cause pneumonia, but most bacterial pneumonias are due to *Streptococcus*. Some strains have developed resistance to antibiotics, so a preventive solution is getting the pneumonia vaccine. This vaccine is given at the same time as the flu shot to high-risk groups such as the elderly. Made from 23 different strains of pneumonia-causing *Streptococcus* bacteria, it's considered a safe and effective solution for preventing pneumonia.

In severe cases of pneumonia, where inflammation causes obstruction of the airways, corticosteroid drugs may be prescribed. There is limited information, however, on the benefits of steroids for lung inflammation associated with viral pneumonia. When faced with the unfamiliar, the medical community turns to the familiar, even if the available choices are clearly ineffective. In the case of steroids, these drugs can seriously dampen the immune system's ability to respond effectively to infection. This is one reason why asthmatics who regularly use oral steroid drugs or inhalers have lowered protection from the influenza vaccine. Also, improper use of steroids may contribute to a relapse of symptoms or to opportunistic bacterial infection that can be worse than the original sickness.

Doctors take that risk, however, because steroids rapidly reduce inflammation. Over the short term, they can save lives. Until more information is available, it is best to avoid using steroid drugs for the treatment of viral pneumonia except in life-threatening situations.

The elderly and people with lung or heart disease are the most likely to develop complications of influenza. Pneumonia is the most serious complication and is uncommon except in susceptible individuals during seasonal influenza outbreaks. Pneumonia starts about five days after onset of the first flu symptoms. Cough worsens and breathing becomes labored. There is persistent or recurring fever and sometimes the person spits up bloody sputum.

Children younger than one year old have a very high risk for pneumonia and other complications, including meningitis and encephalitis (inflammation in the brain and spinal cord). Their immune systems are not strong enough to fend off viral infection. The risk declines as they grow and their immunity becomes stronger, but is still of concern in children aged three to five.

Other complications of flu include inflammation of the small airways of the lungs, bronchitis, sinus infection, and croup caused by swelling of the windpipe, which results in hoarseness and a distinctive barking cough. Symptoms of airway disease and chronic obstructive pulmonary disease can worsen. The virus can cause inflammation and even deterioration of the heart muscle and other muscles in the body. Persistent fatigue can be troublesome for weeks, months, or longer after flu symptoms are gone.

3
Masters of Mutation

How Viruses Evolve and Make Us Sick

WHAT'S A VIRUS?

A virus is essentially a spherical protein envelope or coating containing a set of genetic material that constitutes its code of biological behavior. Microscopically small, 1/10,000 of a millimeter in diameter, viruses have the potential to infect everything from bacteria to whales.

Composed of a nucleic acid core of either RNA or DNA, but not both, the protein coat protects a virus during its journey from host to host and during cell-hopping within the host. Higher organisms, as in human cells, contain both sets of genetic material. RNA viruses outnumber DNA types. The infecting virus has to highjack genetic material inside the host cell's nucleus, the command center of the cell, in order to replicate.

Essentially, viruses are intracellular parasites. They have no life of their own outside a living cell. It's because of this trait that scientists find it hard to tell if viruses are alive at all.

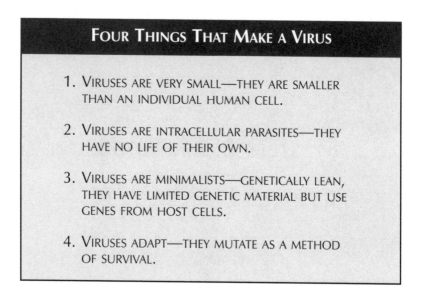

FOUR THINGS THAT MAKE A VIRUS

1. VIRUSES ARE VERY SMALL—THEY ARE SMALLER THAN AN INDIVIDUAL HUMAN CELL.

2. VIRUSES ARE INTRACELLULAR PARASITES—THEY HAVE NO LIFE OF THEIR OWN.

3. VIRUSES ARE MINIMALISTS—GENETICALLY LEAN, THEY HAVE LIMITED GENETIC MATERIAL BUT USE GENES FROM HOST CELLS.

4. VIRUSES ADAPT—THEY MUTATE AS A METHOD OF SURVIVAL.

Amidst the many unsolved mysteries of viral biology, one thing is clear scientifically: Viruses mutate. All RNA viruses, which include influenza, tend to have high mutation rates. But influenza virus is the master of mutation. It rearranges itself by an ingenious method called gene swapping.

HOW AND WHY DO VIRUSES MUTATE?

Like all living organisms, viruses have to survive and adapt in an ever-changing biological world of fierce competition. When two or more viruses infect the same animal, or person, they swap genes, recombining to form a stronger, more successful version. Recombination doesn't happen all at once, however. It occurs over time and in different ways.

Inside the body is an incredible environmental soup composed of tissues made up of a quadrillion cells, a hundred trillion bacteria, pounds of proteins, and a vast array of chemicals and hormones that are continuously moving and constantly rubbing into each other. Some fit better together than others, and when they do, they bind and blend. In the process, they exchange genes. By doing so, they adapt to environmental and immune pressures. This is referred to as the theory of random mutation.

Another theory is cumulative error. RNA viruses, such as influenza, have mutation rates more than 10,000 times higher than human cells. After several mutations, genetic changes occur that result in a new strain. The end product can be a very different virus from what it was originally.

Another reason mutations occur is due to immune pressure. This theory assumes that the virus is self-protective and has strategies to avoid detection by the host's immune system and manage to successfully survive within the host. Viruses readily adapt to antiviral drugs, and some drug-resistant variants of bird flu viruses already exist. The human form of H5N1 may become immune to antiviral drugs, creating a super flu.

PASS THE GENES

An influenza virus exchanges information encoded in the genes of its ancestors and relatives. In addition, they are able to use genetic material from other, unrelated organisms. Passing the genes around assures their survival and is the manner by which a super flu strain could develop.

In fact, super bugs already exist, and most are in the hospital. Long-term and widespread use of antibiotics exerts immune pressure on bacteria either to evolve or to become extinct. There are many strains of bacteria that can resist modern antibiotics, with potentially lethal effects for the patients who become infected by them. There is, however, one super bug among them, vancomycin-resistant *Staphylococcus*, that outdoes them all. *Staphylococcus* is so common that most of us have these bacteria in our noses and on our skin, but they can cause infections if they get into wounds.

Super staph is impervious to all antibiotics including the strongest we have, vancomycin. Bacteria have outsmarted the antibiotics; are viruses next?

TO DRIFT OR SHIFT

Antigenic drift, the gradual re-assortment of flu genes, results in the progressive accumulation of mutations. Over time, these small changes make the influenza virus more effective at attaching to and entering human cells. But when more than one type of influenza virus infects the same cell, they strip coatings and swap genes. The result of this rearranging within that cell is a new strain of virus.

At unpredictable intervals, re-assortment can occur at remarkable speed. When what was once thought to be random re-assortment by gene swapping takes place, often occurring between an animal and a human host, a completely new viral strain emerges. Virologists, scientists who study viruses, call this ability of a virus to undergo a major genetic change antigenic shift.

Of the different types of flu viruses, only influenza A undergoes antigenic shift. This trait of rapid mutation makes it difficult to find a universal vaccine, as was done with smallpox. It also provides the potential for pandemics.

HOW EFFICIENT IS INFLUENZA AT MAKING US SICK?

Influenza has been called the last of the great uncontrolled plagues for a very good reason. It spreads readily, enters the body through the air, and attaches easily to sites on the mucous lining of the respiratory tract. It's effective at entering human cells and evolves rapidly in an effort to keep up with our body's immune strategies. It likes crowds and closed spaces, and is most likely to cause sickness during the winter months when people are forced indoors. For the elderly and very young, it can be lethal.

As noted previously, for the first few days after infection there are no symptoms, but the virus is at work, multiplying in geometric proportions. About 24 hours before symptoms develop, you can spread the flu without knowing you're sick. Once you start coughing and have a fever, the virus is already looking for a new host.

With ordinary flu, you remain contagious for about a week from first exposure to shedding of the virus. The contagious period could last longer with pandemic influenza.

Some people get mild forms of the flu or don't develop severe symptoms even though they harbor the virus. Symptom-free or "silent" flu carriers can spread the virus even though not sick enough to be confined to bed. Those with severe symptoms and the highly contagious who fly on an airplane or go to a movie theatre or other public venue can infect scores of people. They are called "super spreaders."

Since heat destroys it, influenza virus likes the cold. It can survive exposure to cool air for weeks. So hours or days after someone infected with the flu has coughed or sneezed into a room, or touched a countertop or doorknob, the virus is there waiting for human contact. It's also possible that it can spread on the wind. Breezy winter or cool spring days can blow viruses into your respiratory tract. The virus can travel in building ventilation systems, making a whole office sick from one contagious person in a different part of the building.

Influenza virus doesn't like sunlight. Another reason why flu is a winter illness is that ultraviolet B wavelengths in sunlight kill influenza virus. The cold, gray days of winter that keep people indoors foster contagion as people brush against each other in elevators and on crowded streets. Flu cases peak when ultraviolet light from the sun is blocked by air pollution from industrial contaminants or from weeks of overcast skies as during the rainy season in the tropics.

THE CHINA CONNECTION

Southern China with its lush green rice paddies, sentinel-shaped hills, abundant rain, and peaceful rivers seems too idyllic to be the breeding ground for countless strains of influenza viruses. But for millennia, this semitropical humid climate with its long growing season has not only been home to hundreds of millions of chickens, ducks, geese, and people, it is also the world's influenza incubator.

Wild birds like gulls, herons, and ducks carry influenza viruses hundreds of miles, mixing strains from one region with those of another. In the cool, moist mornings, Chinese farmers load chickens and Peking ducks into crates and ship them to market in the city, or tying live poultry by their feet in bunches and draping them over bicycles, they pedal the birds into town.

Human and bird viruses have been mixing it up forever in southern China and Southeast Asia where they coexist in conditions highly conducive to breeding disease. Hot, humid, and unsanitary living environments foster microbial growth. People go barefoot in courtyards where chickens peck for insects and litter the ground with their feces. Children bathe in the same irrigation canals and ponds where ducks swim and pigs wallow. At night, animals and birds sleep cheek to beak with humans. Hepatitis, intestinal viruses, and parasitic disease as well as influenza are endemic in China, Southeast Asia, and Indonesia.

Gene swapping is common in nature, but when an animal or human becomes infected by two different influenza strains, the stakes go up. As explained earlier, double infection can result in recombination of genes. Every time another person is infected with the bird flu, the chance of mutation increases and the possibility of a human sickness rises. If antiviral drugs are used indiscriminately and disease resistance develops, a new drug-resistant version may develop. Were it to combine with a lethal gene mutation, we could be faced with a megavirus.

THE ENVIRONMENTAL DIMENSION

A growing number of scientists are concerned that environmental changes and ecological disruption caused by humans are playing a role in the evolution of viruses. Though there's little proof, the list of possible influences is growing and gaining support by scientists and environmentalists. Population explosion is just one of them.

The world is being smothered by people. The more crowded we become, the easier it is for infection to spread, especially in Third World communities where poverty and lack of sanitation are already a breeding ground for disease. There are 25 cities in the world with over 10 million residents and over 400 that have more than one million people. It is not only overcrowding that facilitates the spread of influenza; the massive movement of people, legally and illegally, across borders and within nations by airplane, sea travel, trains, and automobiles may spread a pandemic faster than infected birds can fly.

Another health concern in China is the loss of sunlight caused by burning coal that most Chinese use as fuel in cooking. Much of China is shrouded in gray from air pollution caused by nitrogen dioxide and the problem is getting worse even with cleaner coal technology. In fact, 16 of the world's 20 most polluted cities are in China. Burning trees and grass, as is done in the Brazilian Amazon rainforest to make room for cattle and farming, is causing a brown haze across large regions of the world. When there is not enough sunshine, temperatures drop—a condition favored by influenza virus.

Airborne pollution irritates the lungs, making city dwellers more vulnerable to asthma and respiratory infections. It can also cause genetic defects that increase our vulnerability to disease.

Genetically modified foods that look good on the shelf but are low in essential nutrients comprise another contributing factor to lowered immunity. Packaged and highly processed fast foods are largely devoid of immune-supporting nutrients such as zinc and selenium.

Pandemics arise when a new strain develops and there is a vulnerable population. More than ever before, environmental factors are playing a role in disease evolution. When we factor in immune pressure from the overuse of antiviral drugs, overpopulation, immune deficiency caused by poor diet and malnutrition, air pollution, global travel, and declining sunlight, the conditions seem right for a plague.

4
Prelude to a Pandemic

Why H5N1 Avian Influenza Is So Dangerous

In 1997, a bird flu epidemic emerged in Southeast Asia, killing thousands of chickens and resulting in the slaughter of millions more ordered by governments and the World Health Organization in an attempt to stop it from spreading. The first human case was a three-year-old boy in Hong Kong. The illness was rapid and frightening. Doctors were powerless. In early May 1997, within days after infection, the child was dead.

International health experts sprang into action. What they found was alarming. The disease circulated widely in chickens, ducks, geese, and turkeys. Not long afterward, they found that it was also present in wild birds. This combination of near-universal infection in birds made it impossible to eradicate.

Beating the Flu

Though it started as a bird disease, it can infect humans who come in contact with sick chickens. Once in the body, it has ways of turning off immune mechanisms that signal a viral invasion. Before the immune system is able to respond, it is entrenched in millions of cells. When the immune system recognizes an invasion of the lungs, it explodes by releasing immune chemicals so intense they can overwhelm the body. In some cases, the body kills itself while trying to preserve its own life.

Year after year, in countless numbers of birds, the virus swapped genes and generated myriad variant strains. It was as though it was determined not just to survive, but to win.

In 2001, bird flu cropped up again in Hong Kong markets. It reappeared in 2002. This time Vietnam was hit particularly hard. In 2004, more people were dying from bird flu. By 2005, researchers confirmed cases of human-to-human transmission. Though the virus was still inefficient at spreading among humans, it was learning and it was marching westward. At the end of the year, deaths were reported in Turkey. Europe was next. By winter, the WHO issued a Phase 3 alert, the first stage of a bird flu pandemic. In 2006, it was killing birds and people in Iraq. After SARS in 2003, the 2004 tsunami in the South Pacific, and two of the worst hurricane years in history (2004 and 2005), the world prepared for the worst—a bird flu pandemic.

WHAT'S THE BIRD FLU?

Bird flu is a type of avian influenza (H5N1 avian influenza A) that infects domestic birds such as chickens, ducks, and turkeys. The reservoir for the virus is in the intestines of wild birds, including migratory waterfowl such as ducks, geese, and swans. Serving as a reservoir means the birds carry it but don't get sick, although there have been instances in which flocks of wild birds have died from bird flu, for example, at Qinghai Lake in central China. Wild birds spread the virus in their feces. Mingling with barnyard fowl, wild birds infect domestic ones.

In a commercial chicken-raising facility where tens of thousands of birds are housed closely packed together in cages, the virus can spread like wildfire. The death rate can approach 100 percent.

Once in the domestic bird population, the virus adapts and becomes a deadly influenza, but only in birds. From there it can jump to pigs or people. The bird flu has all the makings of a pandemic virus. It circulates in birds around the world and migratory birds spread it on the wing. Essentially, it's impossible to control.

HOW CAN A CHICKEN VIRUS INFECT PEOPLE?

Usually, bird flu doesn't infect humans. In fact, it shouldn't jump directly from birds to people. But farmworkers who come in contact with infected birds get sick. In the past, to become a human infection, avian viruses used barnyard pigs as a mixing bowl, bridging the biological gap between birds and people. There's no rule that it has to happen this way, however. The virus could use a human as its genetic springboard.

HOW SICK CAN YOU GET?

No one knows when an influenza pandemic will appear, what strain it will be, or how bad it might get. The number of victims it's claiming is increasing, however. Children are hit particularly hard. Fatality among children younger than age 15 infected by bird flu in Thailand has been 89 percent. That's a paralyzing death rate.

Bird flu is unusually aggressive and is considered highly pathogenic. An analysis of the symptoms gives details about what to expect. After infection, it takes several days to a week or more for symptoms to appear. During this time, the virus is actively reproducing and, like a thief, silently learning how to dodge the immune system's defenses.

In birds, incubation (the time between exposure and symptoms) varies from three to seven days. The outcome is sudden death. In humans, the average for incubation is six days, but it can be shorter than that or as long as 17 days. There is no established incubation time for humans.

High fever comes on rapidly. Ordinary influenza-like symptoms follow, including diarrhea, nausea and vomiting, pain in the abdomen and chest, and malaise. But the spectrum of clinical symptoms is broader.

Beating the Flu

As the flu worsens, bleeding from the nose and gums can occur. Watery diarrhea is common and can cause loss of fluids and electrolytes, resulting in extreme weakness. Usually, influenza targets the lungs, but with the bird flu it can bypass the respiratory system and go right to the brain. Two Vietnamese patients had acute encephalitis, a brain inflammation; neither had respiratory symptoms when they went to the hospital.

The bird flu hits the lungs early in the illness. Many patients have difficulty breathing within five days after the first symptoms. Shortness of breath, a hoarse voice, and a crackling sound when inhaling are common first-stage symptoms. As in regular flu, patients have a cough without sputum, but some have blood-tinted secretions. Almost everyone develops viral pneumonia.

That's just the beginning. Deterioration is rapid. On average, it takes only six days after the onset of illness for the development of acute respiratory distress. Breathing becomes impossible. The blood starts to thicken, the heart and kidney falter, and the lungs give out.

HOW FAST DOES BIRD FLU SPREAD?

There are two fundamental things to understand about a super flu pandemic. First, it's a new strain of influenza virus, making it unrecognizable by our immune systems. We will have no immunity against a new influenza strain. Eventually, we'll develop immune recognition and the ability to fight it off, but that can take months or years. Second, nature has designed it to spread from person to person through a cough, sneeze, or touch, making it highly contagious.

Critics among scientists contend that less than a few hundred people have been infected with H5N1. Those that have caught it from people were infected by family members. Since the virus tends to infect the lower lobes of the lungs, they say that it's less likely to spread through coughing. If the virus becomes transmittable between humans, however, it needs only 40 infected people to go global. Within one year, if each infected person spreads the disease to two others, half of the world's population would be infected.

As the virus accelerates, there's little that can stop it. Early treatment with antiviral drugs within the first two days after infection is critical. If the 48-hour window of opportunity is missed, the drugs are not as effective. How many tens of millions of doses of antiviral drugs will it take to stop a pandemic? Will people in the developed nations be willing to give up some of their supply to treat peasants in Vietnam or Laos? Will a safe and effective vaccine come in time?

YEAR OF THE BIRD FLU

In these postmodern global times, scientists are monitoring infection in chicken flocks around the world as well as in hospitalized patients. Reporters are right behind them. It's unlikely, even as governments attempt to prevent mass panic, that the first devastating scenes of a bird flu pandemic won't be televised.

In early 2006, the biochemical and genetic signals were there for a pandemic explosion, with the bird flu able to infect humans as well as birds. The flu hit Iraq hard and moved into Africa. More than 90 people were confirmed dead from the bird flu and 180 million birds were killed by the virus or slaughtered to prevent spread of infection. It was moving faster than expected and showed up in France in February. By the end of May, there were 205 cases worldwide with 113 dead, a 45 percent death rate. In Cambodia and Iraq, 100 percent of those infected died.

New cases were found in the Middle East, Egypt, and Indonesia. Though still not efficient at infecting humans, the virus was learning how to make other mammals sick. Cases of bird flu infection in domestic cats, leopards, tigers, and pigs were increasing. Predictions pointed to bird flu hitting poultry farms in British Columbia and California before summer 2006.

The third warning bell—Phase III—has rung. It's certain that another influenza pandemic will come. The only questions are when and what strain? Will 2007 or later be the year of the bird flu?

Though China has long been considered the incubator of influenza virus and the most likely epicenter of a pandemic avian virus, the unexpected could happen where two or more influenza mutations might arise at the same time and in different places. It's

Beating the Flu

been almost ten years since the first H5N1 bird flu strain appeared in Hong Kong. One of the weaknesses of science is a myopic view that doesn't allow for unpredictable events. In this case, another avian viral lineage could emerge as the pandemic strain. That would not be so good for us if we had spent years developing a vaccine for H5N1 while nature was outflanking science.

The study of H5N1 avian influenza is important. It has exposed human vulnerability, inadequate public health, and lack of preparedness for a pandemic. But modern medical science may be too focused on a magic bullet that when seen through the eyes of tunnel vision could miss the mark entirely.

5
Run and Hide

The Shortcomings of Quarantine and the Importance of Avoidance

The first line of defense against a pandemic is to see it coming. To accomplish that, sophisticated and well-coordinated surveillance systems are in place around the world. Individual rural doctors transmit information of unusual influenza cases to teams of scientific experts and hospital staff, who funnel information about flu-like infections to centers for disease control around the world. In the United States, the Center for Disease Control and Prevention (CDC) is located in Atlanta, Georgia.

Once a pandemic virus is identified, the goal is to contain it. Rapid response is essential. For maximum containment, the virus needs to be detected within 21 days before the first 40 people are infected, and completely contained within 30 days.

Beating the Flu

Though the virus originates in rural China and Southeast Asia, because of the global spread of bird flu there is no telling where a human form will crop up. Under such circumstances, it is not likely that it can be contained in less than a month. Considering the likelihood that a pandemic could start in an area with limited access to modern medical care, experts agree that the current surveillance system is not fast enough to identify and contain a new strain of influenza. Once a pandemic gets going, it will spread rapidly and containing it will be like trying to stop a freight train.

The next line of defense is in the hospital. But only the most severe cases get there. Since early symptoms are similar to ordinary flu, people aren't quick see a doctor. Once a case is hospitalized, things happen fast. Even if it is as far away as Asia, samples of the patient's blood and tissue are rushed to the CDC in the United States. Within 40 hours, experts can tell if it's the bird flu.

As the clock ticks, six hours later scientists can determine the infectiousness of the strain, and within another two days they can tell what antiviral drugs will work against it or reveal if it's resistant so that drugs won't work at all.

That's about five days. Well within the 30-day window. The ideal scenario doesn't usually happen, however. It may have taken several days for the person to be hospitalized. Things can slow down, initial diagnosis can be delayed or wrong, and bureaucracy can paralyze response.

ARE WE READY FOR A PANDEMIC SUPER FLU?

It's not that we don't have a plan. It's that nature is unpredictable. We also tend to overestimate our ingenuity and underestimate nature's power. The triad of unpredictability, under-preparedness, and unexpected flu virulence makes for a pandemic more intense than our defenses.

If we fail to protect ourselves, it will not be because of lack of warning or lack of foresight. It will be because of ineffectiveness in carrying out the plan or because we were unwilling or unable to adapt fast enough to the changing character of a super flu. The virus may simply be more prepared than we are. The signs are already there. A single, pinpointed genetic change can render H5N1 virus completely resistant to the body's antiviral cytokines. This immunological phenomenon, along with lack of initial recognition, makes for a nasty disease.

QUARANTINE

Old-fashioned quarantine, enforced isolation imposed to prevent the spread of contagious disease, could help slow down the rate of infection in some areas where compliance and preparedness are high, as in Western Europe. It many not work as well in Third World countries with high population density, limited medical supplies and infrastructure, and lack of political will. In the United States, where tens of millions of commuters and interstate trucking move goods and people across large distances daily, wide-scale infection could happen before it could be contained. Are experts putting too much hope on quarantine?

The world is a different place from what it was in 1918. With an incubation period of only a few days, people would be getting sicker faster than health services and first responders could cope. An incubation period of one week would be significantly worse. Before any one knew they had the disease and before quarantine could be enforced, other communities and cities would be infected. Quarantine will work if the virus is detected in time, and if it happens in isolated, geographically containable areas. Even then, military personal may be needed to enforce curfews and limit travel. Unfortunately, quarantine is unlikely to work for a bird flu pandemic because the base of infection is worldwide and illness may spring up in multiple locations simultaneously.

ISOLATION

Avoidance, isolation of the most severe cases, rapid identification of super spreaders, and social distancing are more realistic approaches than mass quarantine to slowing the spread of a pandemic.

Sick people, either at home or in the hospital, should be kept apart from healthy people. Disease is spread faster when sick people are clustered in wards. It's not as easy as it sounds because ventilation systems in hospitals can carry viral particles to other parts of the building. Special filtration systems or air purifiers would be required in influenza wards and rooms for the most ill. (One such air sterilization device is Viroxx, manufactured in Germany by Kobra-biotechnic GmbH.)

If a sick individual is spotted before boarding an airplane or entering an office or apartment building, the super-spreader effect could be minimized. The super-spreader effect refers to a single sick person infecting countless others, increasing exponentially the transmission of disease.

We have learned from past pandemics that crowding hastens infection. For this reason, measures to decrease social interaction may become necessary, including school closures, curtailing public gatherings, and resorting to alternative work arrangements such as telecommuting. As infection rates heighten in communities, issues such as care for the sick and getting adequate food and water to them may become logistically challenging, making individual stockpiling of food and water beforehand prudent.

MEETING THE GLOBAL CHALLENGE OF A SUPER FLU PANDEMIC

Skeptics among public health experts say levels of anxiety are rising faster than hospitalized cases of bird flu. Extremists cry that bird flu will be a plague of Biblical proportions. Regardless of opinion, there's one thing for certain: Major trouble is brewing in South Asia. The influenza crucible is about to boil. What are countries doing about it and how are they preparing? Is the level of current efforts commensurate with the scale of the threat we face?

Hong Kong has been the epicenter for previous influenza pandemics and for SARS. It has wealth, highly trained scientists, skilled doctors, sufficient allied healthcare and paramedical workers, and the political will to survive a pandemic. It also has all the right ingredients for an epidemiological disaster. Tens of millions of people pass through its already teaming population each year. Many of its agricultural practices are not modernized. Chickens and ducks are in high demand in busy Cantonese restaurants and hundreds of open-air markets scattered across the city hawk live chickens, fish, and fresh farm produce. Tiny farms crowd the Chinese mainland just over the straits from the islands that make up Hong Kong. All the conditions are in place for mass infection and I've seen them for myself on numerous trips to Hong Kong and China.

To this end, the government of Hong Kong has bought and stockpiled enough antiviral drugs to treat every inhabitant. It also has an abundant supply of traditional Chinese herbal medicine that inhabitants are culturally familiar with and willing to take. Pharmaceutical drugs can be bought without a physician's prescription. Other steps taken include improving marketing practices for live poultry, increasing surveillance, and requiring better sanitation on farms. Culling of diseased birds is mandatory in Hong Kong and farmers are compensated appropriately.

Vietnam, Thailand, and Indonesia, all poorer and larger than Hong Kong, are not as progressive. They argue over culling practices. Impoverished subsistence farmers are reluctant to report sick birds and often eat birds that die. Thailand is a major poultry exporter to Hong Kong and other parts of Asia. Fear of lost revenues often outweighs concern for public health.

Assuming the attitude that there is no room for complacency, the European Union is taking action. As part of a preparedness plan, cooperation between countries and agencies is already occurring, public health systems are being readied, and there is recognition that antiviral drugs are only part of the solution and pose a threat of increasing drug-resistant strains if improperly used.

The United States is inadequately prepared. It's simply too large and too populated to supply everyone with vaccines and antiviral drugs. A good faith plan was initiated in the fall of 2005 to purchase enough antiviral medication to treat 20 million people. What about the remaining 270 million? What about the additional 12 million illegal residents?

The Chinese have a responsibility to cooperate with international health agencies more than they have in the past in order for the world to control avian flu at its source. But will they be willing to be more transparent when international trade is booming and the 2008 Summer Olympics in Beijing is close at hand? China consumes most of its poultry, but the numbers of domestic chickens and ducks are staggering. Despite the odds, in 2004, China adopted a policy of vaccinating all poultry against bird flu. Farming practices in most of China are primitive, however, and contact with animal feces routine.

I went to China several times in the 1980s and 1990s and have experienced the masses of people in Chinese cities. Even the Chinese call it a "sea of humanity." Crowding in Chinese cities is so intense that people walk pressed shoulder to shoulder and ride buses so tightly packed that it is difficult to move to get off. These conditions facilitate the spread of infection. One sneeze could infect every passenger on a city bus.

A few richer and smaller countries are more prepared than others. Most, however, are hampered by lack of resources and infrastructure. Cambodia and Laos, countries contingent to the bird flu epicenter, are lacking in everything needed to contain and treat a super flu outbreak. Many other Asian countries, including the Philippines, are in a similar situation, as are most Caribbean and Latin American countries. The Middle East has nearly no medical infrastructure and is one of the most unprepared regions in the world.

An influenza pandemic is no longer a farfetched speculation. It is not a matter of if, but when. For now, you may not be able to rely completely on governments or agencies to prevent a pandemic or to protect us if one comes. Knowledge is power. You have to learn how to protect yourself and your family by utilizing the power of nature and science.

6
Flu Wars

The Double-Edged Sword of Vaccination and Antiviral Drugs

Conventional modern medicine has two weapons for combating the flu: drugs and vaccines. Antiviral drugs don't actually kill viruses. They only diminish viral replication, which helps lower the infection rate in the body. Other drugs, including antibiotics for opportunistic bacterial infections such as pneumonia and steroids for inflammation, don't always work and can cause serious adverse effects, but are medically necessary components in the influenza-fighting arsenal. None of these drugs is a magic bullet against influenza. At best, these drugs slow the virus down and save lives but they cannot thwart a super flu.

Experts claim that the best chance of slowing down a pandemic flu outbreak rests in rapid immunization of large numbers of people and early treatment with antiviral drugs. That's assuming there are enough shots and pills to go around, the flu strain is not excessively fierce, treatment is effective, and there's a strategy for accomplishing mass immunization and drug dispensing. That's the best-case scenario.

In reality, antiviral drugs won't work and vaccines will be inefficient in a super flu pandemic. Both of these pharmaceutical solutions pose immense risks. Drugs have side effects and cause the virus to become stronger. The result is that they will end up not working at all. Vaccines, if not tested for safety ahead of widespread immunization, may become a health hazard. Vaccine risks include infection from the inoculated virus in susceptible individuals, autoimmune reactions, and damage to the nervous system from toxic substances in the vaccine.

In this chapter, you'll find a discussion on the benefits and risks of the limited number of medications we have to fight the flu. I'm not opposed on principle to vaccination and the use of antiviral drugs or antibiotics. For me, it's not a philosophical debate. If anything, I lean toward an integrative philosophy of medical care. Because a pandemic threat is potentially overwhelming, I'm concerned about what's clinically the safest and most effective means of prevention and treatment, and without adverse reactions. It's not enough to fight it; we must beat the flu.

VACCINES

Even if we had a safe and effective vaccine, it would not prevent the global spread of the flu. Using current flu vaccines as a model, we see that, though helpful some of the time in reducing the severity of infection, they do not eliminate widespread sickness nor eradicate the disease. At best, they reduce symptom severity and shorten the duration of sickness by a day or two. Not a great margin.

Each year, new flu vaccine has to be made, and because influenza A virus is so cunning, and because no one knows which of the many diverse strains will hit in any one season, three different flu strains are combined in one cocktail. Guessing wrong renders it useless.

To be effective, the match between vaccine and disease must be close, if not exact. The closer the match, the better the immune system can recognize infection and defend against the virus. To match it exactly, however, which is our best bet for an effective vaccine, the specific disease strain must be in circulation. In other words, once the pandemic gets going, we can start making vaccine. From start to finish, that would take six months. Then it has to be distributed and shots given to people. The H5N1 virus mutates rapidly, however, so even with a good match, the strain could change its genetic code and outflank our immunological strategies.

To make a vaccine stop a flu pandemic, there has to be enough supply and it has to be safe and tested, not only on laboratory rats, but also on humans. The obstacles to making an adequate number of doses are immense and involve decision-making in politics, technology, science, medicine, and business. They include ethical issues like who will get flu shots when there are not enough, and whether one country will share its supply with another.

Trying to slow down a pandemic is like trying to turn around a giant freighter. It takes time and room to maneuver. But the flu is not a giant ship at sea. It's more like a fast-moving storm. A vaccination campaign might help. But experts contend that a sizable percentage of all people will need to be inoculated in order to lessen a pandemic's force.

Scientists and governments are not waiting. In 2004, H5N1 seed virus from a Vietnamese bird flu victim was distributed to research centers with the goal of creating a vaccine. Preliminary results from clinical trials indicate that the developed vaccine would be partially effective against avian influenza in humans. But no one knows what amount is needed to protect a human adult. Some studies suggest that it could take eight to ten times more than needed in a conventional flu vaccine. If this were the case, 20 million doses, the number the American government wants, would only yield two to three million effective doses.

One drug company, GlaxoSmithKline, started trials on a H5N1 vaccine in the spring of 2006 in Germany and Belgium using an adjuvant to enhance its effect. Adjuvant technology means a lower amount of vaccine is needed per dose. That might increase the number of doses available. The vaccine still has to be effective and safe, however. Initial results from the trials, designed to test safety and measure immune response, are expected by the flu season of 2006–2007.

There's another concern. Since no one will have built up immunity to a new strain, for the vaccine to be effective people will need two shots. The first one is a primer to get the immune system geared up. About four weeks later, the second shot or booster is given. After that, it takes eight months for the human immune system to develop immunity. By that time, a pandemic flu could circle the globe.

Scientists have other tricks such as reverse genetics and recombination, in which an entire library of new viruses is made in the lab with characteristics of a wild virus. Vaccines made in this way contain live viruses (conventional flu vaccines are made from dead ones) and are administered in a nasal spray. Needle-free vaccination is appealing to many people, but is it safe to spray massive amounts of live laboratory viruses up your nose?

If an influenza pandemic occurs in 2012, we might be ready. If a fast-moving super flu occurs before then, we won't be prepared. Even if we have a close match, vaccine manufacturers can't produce enough dosages fast enough.

Vaccines will be controlled by governments, with key leaders first in line for inoculation, followed by medical workers and first responders such as firefighters, then workers in drug and vaccine factories, and those at most risk such as pregnant women, infants, and the elderly. Who will make the decision about who gets vaccinated after that? What agency will determine if a vaccine is safe for mass vaccination?

The answer is frightening. In November 2005, the U.S. Senate reviewed a bill to create a biodefense agency that could operate in secrecy, have no accountability, and enforce medical treatment on every citizen. The new governmental arm would be called the Biomedical Advanced Research and Development Agency (BARDA). Its purpose is to develop countermeasures against an act of bioterrorism or natural disease outbreaks such as a flu pandemic. But opponents call it the creation of a medical Gestapo. Any adverse consequences caused by drugs or vaccines used to prevent or treat pandemic flu would be exempt from legal recourse or compensation. Experimental drugs could be released before being fully tested and orphan drugs, medications intended for an entirely different condition, could be used even if considered dangerous.

Let's keep things in perspective. In the 1970s, the success of massive immunization against smallpox and polio was heralded as a major human victory over viruses. But that's only partially true. Public health measures and improved nutrition helped as much to control disease spread. Smallpox vaccine works, but, unfortunately, other viruses aren't as easy. Countless influenza strains circulate at the same time and each is constantly evolving, some at an unbelievable pace. A super flu strain would be nearly impossible to pin down.

Evolutionary biologists have suggested that perhaps there is an ecological need for viruses, including smallpox, as a means of keeping our immune systems strong. When humans tamper with millions of years of natural evolution, we may not realize the repercussions for generations.

Reverberations still ring in scientific halls about the wisdom, or lack of foresight, of mass immunization. In 1976, an army private became sick with a mysterious strain of swine flu. Pigs had been infected with influenza before, but only rarely did it pass on to humans. But government scientists weren't taking any chances. The fervor of the moment, political pressures, and fear of a repeat of the 1918 influenza pandemic spurred them on and the United States launched a massive immunization program.

This involved purchasing tens of millions of fertile chicken eggs and then cultivating the viruses needed to make vaccine under the supervision of the Bureau of Biologics. The goal: Vaccinate every American. Ten days after the first round of vaccinations, the deaths started. Some people dropped dead within minutes after inoculation. Then a rare nervous system disease, Guillain-Barré syndrome, developed in some who got the shot. In all, 40 million people were vaccinated for swine flu. As a consequence, about 70 people died and hundreds developed Guillain-Barré syndrome. When no pandemic emerged, the litigation began. In the end, 3,917 claims were filed. People had been killed and crippled, and the survivors were angry that scientists, medical doctors, vaccine manufacturers, and politicians hadn't been wiser.

FROM HEN TO HOSPITAL

The process of making vaccines is more like something from centuries ago than that of modern science. Though robots are used to mechanize the process, individual fertile chicken eggs are required to grow the virus. When there is enough virus inside the egg, it's extracted and chemically processed for key proteins, called antigens, that stimulate the human immune system to make immune chemicals, called antibodies, against the invading virus. It's a slow, tedious, time-consuming process, requiring about six months from inoculated egg to shot.

Complications don't end with logistical delays, shortages, and a cumbersome laboratory process. Inefficiency also plays a role. Avian influenza H5 strains grow poorly in eggs. Each batch produces much less antigen than when making a vaccine for ordinary flu. Four eggs are needed to make one to two conventional flu shots. That's four billion fertile eggs to vaccinate less than one-quarter of the world's population. But would enough chickens free of bird flu lay enough eggs?

Because the risk of a pandemic is so imminent, the danger so great, and the profits for a new vaccine so high, scientists are feverishly working to develop egg-independent shots. One alternative is a recombination system that constructs a variety of viral genetic strains including possible antigenic drift types. This method produces many more viruses than can be made in eggs. It has the further advantage of avoiding the use of eggs laid by chickens potentially infected with bird flu virus. Still, at least one booster shot is required with recombinant vaccines.

Recombinant vaccines have been developed for other viral diseases (e.g., Marburg virus, a relative of Ebola that causes hemorrhagic fever), but only in animal models, not in people. Such vaccines have the ability to confer immunity but also stimulate the immune system to produce more interferon and cytotoxic T (CD8) cells, both necessary for a strong viral defense against the flu. Though all the details have yet to be worked out for these novel vaccine techniques, not to mention how much it will cost, recombinant vaccines could be a step in the right direction.

If a bird flu vaccine were to become available and needed on short notice, it would be impossible to know all the risks associated with vaccination, especially of adverse events that may occur in the future.

Our common biology may bond us humans in the event of a pandemic super flu. When one is vulnerable, we all are susceptible. Science needs to be harnessed effectively. Governments need to be objective and free from the pressures of the commercial interests of pharmaceutical industry giants. Vaccines need to assure personal safety and be delivered in a timely manner. Distribution must be ethical and compassionate. And the vaccines must be effective.

ANTIVIRAL DRUGS

Antiviral drugs, compared to antibiotics, are relatively new to the clinical scene. Though they are considered complementary to vaccines in the treatment of influenza, many doctors don't have experience with them.

Taken within 48 hours from the onset of symptoms, prescription antiviral drugs shorten the period of illness, reduce the severity of the symptoms, and lessen complications. That's the good news. But clinical data are limited regarding utilization of these drugs with H5N1 influenza and only preliminary laboratory data indicate that, if the drugs are administered early, the avian influenza virus will succumb.

Oseltamivir phospate (Tamiflu) and zanamivir (Relenza): These drugs may reduce the severity of symptoms and save lives, but only if taken in the first 48 hours after infection. There are not enough supplies to go around, however. Governments and individuals are already stockpiling supplies of Tamiflu, the preferred drug of the two because it comes in a pill, whereas Relenza is a powder that needs to be inhaled. But there's concern that personal stockpiles will be used improperly and lead to Tamiflu-resistant influenza.

When used correctly, and barring drug resistance, these drugs can reduce the spread of infection and possibly slow down a fast-moving pandemic. Tamiflu is considered the more effective and easiest to take. There appears to be no greater benefit from taking a 150 mg dosage versus 75 mg.

Though both drugs may reduce the risk of respiratory complications of the flu, adverse effects can result from taking them. Possible side effects include nausea and vomiting, as well as skin rashes, dizziness, and tightening of the airways. Pregnant women should avoid taking these drugs. Interactions with other drugs are considered unlikely according to current data, but they have not been used extensively or long enough to know all the risks.

Ribavirin: A broad-spectrum antiviral with many different trade and generic names, ribavirin has been around for several decades. It's used in the treatment of hepatitis C in combination with interferon and was used extensively during the SARS epidemic. SARS patients died despite its use, however, and some recovered who never took ribavirin. It can cause anemia and reduce calcium and magnesium levels in the body. Other side effects include mood changes including severe depression, skin rashes, eye inflammation, and breathing difficulties. Ribavirin has activity against influenza A virus but has not been well tested against the H5N1 avian influenza. Given its lack of effectiveness in the treatment of SARS and its high side-effect profile, it's an unlikely candidate for use during a bird flu pandemic.

Amantadine (Symmetrel) and rimantadine (Flumadine): Once helpful for ordinary influenza, these antiviral drugs are no longer considered useful. The problem with them is that the virus quickly adapts and they become ineffective. They are also toxic to the body. Of the two, amantadine is the more effective, especially if you haven't been vaccinated against the flu. Common side effects include nausea, constipation, and loss of appetite. Serious complications can also develop, including hearing loss, anxiety, confusion, insomnia, hallucinations, and blurred vision.

Antibiotics: Antibiotics kill bacteria. They are useless against influenza virus. Though they have no value in the treatment of viruses, millions of unnecessary doses of antibiotics are prescribed every year. They have great value, however, in the treatment of severe complications of the flu when these are caused by bacterial infection. Judicious use is essential because many bacteria are antibiotic resistant.

The most commonly used antibiotics for respiratory complications of the flu such as sinusitis and bronchitis are amoxicillin, trimethoprim-sulfamethoxazole (Bactrim and Septra), and doxycycline. Newer broad-spectrum antibiotics are used as second-line defense when these don't work and include clarithromycin (Biaxin) and levofloxacin (Levaquin). Side effects of antibiotics are notorious and include nausea, vomiting, diarrhea, and allergic symptoms including rashes. A pre-existing yeast infection usually gets worse when the person takes antibiotics. Antibiotics can also cause a serious type of colitis, pseudomembranous colitis, which is difficult to eradicate.

Usually antibiotics are taken in pill form, but in severe infections you'll need a shot or an intravenous drip for the medication to be effective. Also, more than one antibiotic may be necessary to get an infection under control. Prescribing antibiotics is best left to a knowledgeable doctor.

Corticosteroids: Steroids reduce inflammation. They can save lives when administered correctly. Overuse of corticosteroid drugs (Cortisol, Dexamethesone, Methylprednisone, Prednisone), however, poses serious danger to the body. They can suppress the immune system to such a degree that other infections can take hold. Side effects include increased appetite and nervousness. Steroids can also aggravate diabetes and glaucoma. Long-term use can cause osteoporosis. Changes in metabolism can take place from chronic steroid use, causing a condition called Cushing's syndrome. Features of this disease include abdominal obesity, a moon-shaped face, and a "buffalo hump" on the upper back. Steroids are a dangerous class of drugs and should be used only when absolutely necessary and as prescribed by a knowledgeable doctor.

Vaccination against pneumonia: Since pneumonia is the most serious fatal complication of influenza, prevention and effective treatment are essential. Antibiotics are the main line of treatment but are useless for viral pneumonia. They are effective only against bacterial pneumonia. And though they work much of the time, they have potential adverse effects. All benefits from chemical drugs come with risks. The question is: Is the benefit greater than the risk? Given that one of the leading causes of death in the United States is prescription drugs, more and more medical doctors are siding with more moderate use of dangerous medications in order to reduce danger to the patient. The pneumonia vaccine, for example, is effective and a much better preventive solution than taking antibiotics after the fact; the latter may not work and could cause adverse effects.

Is There Anything Else?

Allopathic medicine and the pharmaceutical industry have little else to offer for the treatment of influenza. There are unapproved drugs and off-label use of current drugs, however, and they should be seriously investigated and evaluated. The problem with governments and big pharmaceutical companies is that they promote what's in their best interest. What's best for the individual, the general population, and society are not first priority. Many valuable medications, both pharmaceutical drugs and natural remedies, are ignored if they compete with existing patented drugs or are not seen as immensely profitable. Here are some potentially valuable drugs being developed by small companies.

Peramivir, a drug in the same class of antiviral medications as Tamiflu, blocks the viral life cycle and is being tested for single intravenous use against influenza virus. Results so far look favorable, but peramivir is associated with the same concern as all antiviral drugs: Widespread use could trigger drug resistance. First developed in 1987, it was poorly absorbed by the body when given as a pill and was therefore not effective. Researchers investigating its effectiveness when introduced directly into a vein and possibly as an intramuscular injection are finding that this seems to work. When the body is overwhelmed with infection, drugs tend to be more effective when they are introduced directly into the bloodstream. Peramivir deserves another look.

Redesigning and recycling existing drugs is another option. A synthetic version of Tamiflu is under development in Japan. If ready in time, it could meet the huge demand for global stockpiles. Drugs used to normalize excessive immune reactions, which occur in SARS and bird flu victims, may be adapted to treat the over-response of harmful immune messengers like tumor necrosis factor and interleukin-6. When in excess, these substances cause massive inflammation and can lead to organ failure and death. Swedish researchers have proposed using drugs such as etoposide to kill excess immune cells in order to save lives in the most severe cases.

Nature is an excellent source of antiviral medicines. For example, Tamiflu is derived from the star anise plant. One drug company, Aphios, is looking for new influenza drugs in plants and marine microorganisms. A French Canadian company, Replicor, is working on a broad-spectrum antiviral drug that has both preventative and therapeutic use. Given the resilience of influenza virus, having alternative drugs is an important aspect of pandemic preparedness.

OVERKILL

The germs might well win. Already, we've seen the consequences of overuse of antibiotics and antimalarial drugs. Antibiotic-resistant tuberculosis, mefloquine and artemisinin combination therapy for the treatment of malaria, and antibiotic-resistant *Staphylococcus* strains in hospitals are but a few cases of the germs winning. Indeed, drug resistance is becoming routine.

The World Health Organization is concerned that resistance to drugs is reaching a crisis point. All major life-threatening infections including tuberculosis, pneumonia, malaria, and diarrheal disease and many common infections such as sinusitis and bladder infections are already impervious to antibiotics.

Though bacteria lead the way, viruses are right behind. Two

influenza-fighting drugs don't work any longer, and there are resistant strains of HIV and hepatitis. When more drugs are given, resistance increases. Bugs, it turns out, are very good at dodging drugs.

Already, the H5N1 virus is resistant to the older antiviral drugs amantidine and ramantidine. These are unlikely to work against an emerging human avian flu strain. Drug resistance to the touted anti-flu drug oseltamivir has been reported and investigation is under way to determine just how widespread drug resistance is. But clinical data are spotty. And it's always possible that genetic reassortment could produce a super strain that is invulnerable to any of our few remaining antiviral medications.

Antiviral drugs are not the solution to a bird flu pandemic. Stockpiling and the potential overuse and inappropriate treatment with antiviral drugs could easily lead to a drug-resistant strain far worse than the original one. Though exerting some effects on management of symptoms, these drugs won't prevent infection and don't dramatically reduce the viral load in your body. Overestimating the ability of these antiviral drugs to treat sickness and control an influenza plague provides a false sense of security. In my clinical opinion, overreliance on an exclusively pharmacological approach to pandemic influenza is dangerous and unwise.

7
Lessons from SARS

What We Learned from an Epidemic

In the spring of 2003, a new virus was killing people in Asia. In response to a mysterious respiratory tract infection, which was to become known as severe acute respiratory syndrome (SARS), public health experts converged on Hong Kong and China. SARS causes a type of viral pneumonia with symptoms much like influenza: fever, dry cough, and shortness of breath. Death results from progressive respiratory failure. And like a cold or flu, it's spread by drops of moisture coughed or sneezed into the air. The world was on edge.

In a matter of a few months, SARS arrived in Stockholm and Toronto by airplane. The Canadian government set up a SARS war room and got ready to confront the worst. But neither government nor public health officials were prepared. One Canadian physician said it was like trying to invent a bucket after the fire had started.

At final count, Hong Kong had 1,755 reported cases. Mainland China, far from candid about its internal affairs and accused of grossly under-reporting the number of cases, had an official 5,327. The total number of reported cases worldwide between November 2002 and July 2003, a period of eight months, was 8,096, of which 774 died. That's a death rate of 9.6 percent. In Hong Kong, the death rate was 17 percent. Unofficially, it could have been higher.

What made it headline news? Why were governments scared? What lessons did we learn from SARS that could help us prepare for an influenza pandemic?

FROM PLATE TO PEOPLE

SARS started in wild palm civet cats, a distant vegetarian cousin of house cats but with a masked face like a raccoon. A delicacy in southern China, where people are accused of eating everything with four legs but the kitchen table, the animal virus readily jumped to humans who handled and ate the meat. From there, it genetically reorganized itself into a highly contagious strain of a previously common virus and then spread from person to person. Usually, viruses require an intermediate mixing bowl such as pigs before becoming a human illness. This time it went right from plate to people, and if it happened once, it could happen again.

What's astonishing is that a virus that was known to be one of the causes of the common cold became a killing machine. Two to ten percent of colds are caused by coronaviruses, the family of viruses to which the SARS virus belongs. Coronaviruses are named after a crownlike halo of protein spikes, which help them to attach to their host cells. But in this instance, instead of the sniffles, the viruses latched on and the victim was dead within a few weeks.

In an unprecedented effort, scientists worked around the clock to come up with the genetic code of the new disease. While SARS gained speed, they studied its patterns and looked for weaknesses in its defenses. Within a few weeks, two independent teams from

Canada and the United States sequenced the entire genome.

While researchers worked on cracking its code, doctors and nurses treated patients with antiviral medicines, antibiotics, and steroids. Still, patients suffered and died. None responded dramatically to pharmaceutical drugs. Fear of a deadly drug-resistant virus running rampant heightened the scare. People in Beijing panicked and exited the city by the thousands.

Then, surprisingly, SARS lost momentum and faded out before becoming a pandemic. Why did it slow down and all but disappear? Should it return to haunt us, will we be ready next time?

ALL IN THE MIX

Virologists believe that, for a new strain to emerge, it has to mix different types of virus from the same family in an intermediate host. Historically, pigs served this purpose when they caught a chicken flu and a human flu at the same time. SARS showed us beyond a doubt, however, and there is evidence that the 1918 Spanish flu was similar, that viral respiratory tract infections can start in an animal, jump directly to people, and mutate without an intermediate host into a highly lethal disease.

The SARS virus was immunologically distinct. As a new infection, the human immune system wasn't prepared to cope with it. To make matters worse, the virus mutated rapidly and unpredictably; so even if you got sick and recovered, you could become infected again. To your immune system, it was an entirely new infection and once again it was not ready to fight it. The wily virus didn't stop there. Rapidly mutating strains made the disease more severe; such viruses tend to be more deadly. It also displayed an ability to outsmart antiviral drugs.

Since the virus caused severe inflammation of the lungs and there was no immunity against it, a deadly form of pneumonia developed and patients suffocated. Combination therapy with the antiviral drug ribavirin and steroids was used to treat it. In up to 20 percent of cases, however, the drugs didn't work because the virus was resistant to its effects. The U.S. Army Medical Research Institute of Infectious Diseases at Fort Detrick in Maryland tested more than 300,000 compounds in the hope of finding a cure for SARS. None worked.

A complicating factor in treating SARS in this manner was that the high dosage of steroids used to treat the inflammation also suppressed immune function, with the result of prolonging the illness. Not a promising scenario for patients.

The SARS epidemic demonstrated the futility of the steroid approach. The use of steroids to treat SARS began in China. On December 22, 2002, Dr. Zhong Nanshan, director of the Guangzhou Institute of Respiratory Diseases, saw a 41-year-old patient with severe pneumonia that wasn't responding to antibiotics. At the time, no one knew that the man was one of the first cases of SARS.

Determining that the pneumonia was caused by the patient's own immune system reacting to an exotic pathogen, Dr. Zhong prescribed corticosteroids to control the inflammation. Within days, the opaque haze that clouded x-rays of the man's lungs began to dissipate and his breathing became more relaxed. Dr. Zhong endorsed big doses, known as "pulses" of steroids, for patients in grave condition. Though the treatment was far from perfect, he concluded that the majority of patients showed improvement. His method for treating SARS caught on and was used aggressively in Beijing. To prevent suffocation from inflamed lungs, steroids flowed by intravenous drips into the veins of thousands of patients.

It wasn't until after they were released from the hospital that a debilitating and often irreversible bone disease called avascular necrosis struck. The bones of the people treated for SARS with high doses of corticosteroids were falling apart.

In Beijing, orthopedic surgeons estimate that a third of the city's 2,500 SARS patients suffered from avascular necrosis. It has long been known that steroids can lead to avascular necrosis. Symptoms typically begin with stiffness or pain in the hip, knee, ankle, or shoulder joints, and can culminate in the crumbling of bones, requiring grafts or joint replacements. Even in milder cases, people can end up with crippling arthritis.

If such adverse outcomes are well known in medicine, why did doctors prescribe high doses of steroids to mass groups of people? If this condition occurred from drug misuse, what other side damage may have happened? These questions may never be answered, but the excessive use of corticosteroids to treat SARS is clearly a warning. Because of such tragic adverse effects, high-dose steroids should be reserved for the most serious cases.

The Chinese Medicine Experience

Ancient Chinese healers studied febrile diseases and epidemics as early as the sixth century. The world's first record of vaccination against smallpox occurred in China in 1562, more than two centuries before it was used in Europe. The concept of disease prevention dates back even further.

From the perspective of traditional Chinese medicine (TCM), prevention means strengthening the body's ability to resist disease and revitalizing the individual's constitution. Fortifying the body begins with lifestyle and dietary changes, rest and sleep, exercise, and drinking herbal decoctions made from astragalus, ginseng root, and other immune-boosting herbs.

Early recognition of symptoms and immediate treatment are also part of the strategy of TCM. First lines of defense are drawn at the surface of the body on the skin, in the muscles, and via acupuncture meridians. Second lines are in the throat, nose, and upper airways. Invading diseases such as the influenza virus are best repelled while the infection is still incipient and hasn't penetrated deeper into the body. When it does, lines of battle are redrawn in the lungs, and even deeper defenses are established in the organs and blood. Different herbal formulas are matched to specific lines of defense.

Epidemic influenza-like respiratory tract disease, which includes SARS, is called *wen bing* and is well known to traditional Chinese doctors. Two ancient formulas, *Sang Ju Yin* (Morus and Chrysanthemum Combination) and *Yu Ping Feng San* (Jade Screen Wind Powder), were in short supply in Hong Kong during the SARS outbreak. In Beijing, an adaptation of a traditional formula nicknamed *Ba Wei* (Eight Ingredients) was in demand. A preparation made by Tong Ren Tang, China's most prestigious herbal manufacturer and pharmacy, *Ba Wei* formula is used in the initial stage of cold and flu. At the peak of the SARS crisis in Hong Kong, herbal preparations were given free of charge to 3,160 at-risk hospital workers. None of them became sick.

But can chunks of tree bark, yellowish slivers of dried roots, and flower buds that look more like yard rakings than medicine treat severe acute viral infection? Hundreds of millions of Chinese attest that traditional herbal remedies work. When scientifically scrutinized, the answer lies in what these plant parts do in the body.

Some, such as astragalus, stimulate the production of interferon, an important immunological first line against viruses. Compounds that lower fever are found in isatis leaf and are useful during the initial acute stage. Many herbs, such as andrographis, have antiviral activity and slow the rate of infection in the body. Researchers at the University of Frankfurt in Germany have shown that glycyrrhizin, a compound derived from licorice root with anti-inflammatory effects and originally a part of the Chinese medicine chest, killed the SARS virus. A nontoxic medicine when used properly, and already employed for hepatitis C virus, glycyrrhizin was the only medication that worked, but only at very high doses. Unfortunately, at these levels, it caused side effects, including elevated blood pressure.

SARS was a serious disease and proved difficult to treat. Drugs had little effect. And though in later studies herbs were shown to be no more effective than ribavirin and steroids, which were ineffective, they were not scientifically proven to be less effective than drugs. In fact, they improved symptoms and quality of life in hospitalized SARS patients and may even have helped shorten the length of time the patient spent in the hospital. Several herbs improved absorption of fluid from the lung so patients didn't suffocate on their own secretions, and others helped lower inflammation so fewer steroids were needed.

In China, where herbal preparations are used extensively and Western and Eastern medicine is integrated in hospitals, the death rate was seven percent. Among those that were already severely ill and treated exclusively with Western drugs, the death rate was an astonishing 47 percent. In comparison, among the most ill who were treated with a combination of Western and Eastern medicine, the death rate was 15 percent. Research suggests that Chinese herbs have immune-regulatory effects that contributed to saving peoples lives.

In the absence of effective antiviral drugs and vaccines, viral infections that cause deadly respiratory tract diseases like SARS and avian influenza should be taken seriously. Alternatives including natural medicines may be important in the prevention and treatment of these diseases and should be investigated thoroughly.

WHAT DID WE LEARN?

The economic repercussions of the SARS outbreak cost the world 150 billion dollars. Airports closed and travel advisory warnings were in effect, paralyzing international travel. Hotels faced massive cancellations. Retail sales plummeted, and meetings and concerts were

---

SIX THINGS WE LEARNED FROM SARS THAT COULD HELP BEAT PANDEMIC INFLUENZA

1. A LETHAL HUMAN VIRUS CAN JUMP DIRECTLY FROM AN ANIMAL VIRUS.

2. A COMMON VIRUS CAN MUTATE INTO A KILLER.

3. IN A FAST-MOVING PLAGUE, THERE'S NO TIME TO COME UP WITH A VACCINE.

4. ANTIVIRAL DRUG RESISTANCE DEVELOPS SO QUICKLY THAT PHARMACEUTICAL DRUGS HAVE NO EFFECT.

5. STEROID DRUGS POSE IMMENSE RISK WHEN USED IMPROPERLY.

6. CHINESE HERBAL MEDICINE MAY HAVE HAD THE SAME EFFECT AS DRUGS, OR BETTER, ON ALL BUT THE MOST SEVERE CASES.

cancelled across Asia. Stock markets wavered. While the global economy tottered, healthcare systems were strained, and medical insurance claims skyrocketed, but pharmaceutical sales boomed. Manufacturers of face masks, hand sanitizers, and emergency supplies couldn't keep pace with demand.

An influenza pandemic would be far worse. It could cost 800 billion, crush many small economies, cripple some countries for decades to come, and all but collapse global trade.

SARS was the first new virus of the twenty-first century. Though many mysteries remain, we learned that timely warning can avert widespread infection. Science is capable, but public health measures need upgrading. Medicine is behind as well. In fact, it may be operating according to an outdated paradigm. A flu pandemic will occur and SARS was the warning shot.

PART II

THE SOLUTION

Natural Prescriptions for Survival

8
Viral Immunity

Enhance Your Body's Defenses against the Flu

Diseases evolve. Our immune systems evolve too and respond to infection in remarkable ways. Most of the time, our systems counter infection with astonishing efficacy. In fact, we get sick far less often than we should considering the number of exposures we have daily to bacteria, parasites, fungi, insect bites, and viruses. But the wager between victim and victor can be high.

A virus can infect you only if you are vulnerable to it. The immune system has a way of cataloging viruses so after the first infection it knows exactly how to respond. In the case of a new strain of influenza, such as H5N1, however, we are all susceptible because our immune systems can't recognize it and initiate the appropriate immune response fast enough.

Beating the Flu

Reducing vulnerability is necessary for beating the flu; strengthening your viral immunity is essential. Influenza pandemics end not because of the effectiveness of drugs or vaccines, but because our immune systems learn to outsmart the virus. Survival depends ultimately not on drugs but on our own viral immunity.

WHAT'S VIRAL IMMUNITY?

Viral immunity is the ability of the immune system to detect, respond to, defend against, neutralize the spread and prevent replication of, viruses in the body, and eliminate them. The immune system has evolved a network of antiviral processes and a diversity of immunological strategies to protect us from infection. Still, stealth viruses can enter our cells undetected and set up control centers, using our own genetic material to run their operation and make us sick.

A viral infection is an invasion. The immune system goes into action as soon as it recognizes invading viruses in the body. Viral-infected cells send out a distress call that induces specialized genes to signal the release of interferon, the body's first-line defense mechanism against viruses. Programmed cell death switches are turned on, signals are sent to inflammatory chemicals, and cell stress alarms are activated.

The virus fights back. It blocks viral immune responses by cutting links to its control center and disrupting communication lines between interferon and immune cells. H5N1 avian influenza has taken it a step further. By switching a single amino acid in its molecular structure, it becomes completely resistant to the body's own best viral-fighting chemical, interferon. Scientists are baffled by this development, but be assured that our immune systems are at work finding a way to beat the flu.

If the immune system outperforms the strategy of the virus, it blocks viral replication and thereby controls the viral hordes that cause infection. In the process, it learns another facet of viral strategy, creates memory cells, and encodes this information in its genetic library under viral-countering methods, so the next time it's ready.

TEST YOUR VIRAL IMMUNITY

- ❏ I GET FEWER THAN TWO COLDS OR ORDINARY FLU A YEAR.

- ❏ I DON'T HAVE ALLERGIES OR ASTHMA, AND I DON'T HAVE LUNG DISEASE.

- ❏ I AM BETWEEN THE AGES OF 15 AND 50.

- ❏ I TAKE ANTIOXIDANT VITAMINS (INCLUDING VITAMIN C AND E) AND MINERALS DAILY.

- ❏ I EXERCISE AT LEAST THREE TIMES A WEEK.

- ❏ I EAT AT LEAST 4–5 SERVINGS OF FRESH FRUIT AND VEGETABLES DAILY.

- ❏ I DRINK FEWER THAN 2–4 GLASSES OF ALCOHOL EACH WEEK.

- ❏ I DON'T SMOKE.

- ❏ I GET 7–9 HOURS OF SLEEP EACH NIGHT.

- ❏ I DON'T HAVE A HIGH STRESS LIFESTYLE.

Score Yourself: Each question to which you answer yes is worth 10 points. 100 points is excellent. 80–90 is very good. 70 is just passing. 50–60 points means you need a viral immunity workout. Less than 50 means your viral immunity is low and you may be highly susceptible to pandemic influenza. Get started on a serious plan to enhance your viral immunity.

Adapted from material found in *Viral Immunity: A 10-Step Plan to Enhance Your Immunity against Viral Disease Using Natural Medicines* (Hampton Roads, 2002).

Beating the Flu

The immune system can be savage, however. If it recognizes that the virus is resistant to its immune strategy, it can mount a cytokine firestorm, releasing massive levels of interferon and tumor necrosis factor, another important virus-fighting chemical, against every infected cell in the body. Unfortunately, in doing so, it damages sensitive tissue, sets off inflammation, destroys important organs such as the brain and liver, and can kill the individual. It's like programmed death—nature's safeguard for uncontrolled infection.

Viral immunity is a complex process. It involves countless cells and a coordinated effort that starts at the port of entry, the mucous membranes of the respiratory tract. Optimal prevention would stop the virus from attaching to mucous membranes in the eyes, nose, throat, and airways. Though the immune system maintains specialized cells at the mucosal lining, like sentries at the gates of the castle, some viruses get past them and gain entry.

Burrowing its way into the tissue and later entering the bloodstream, the virus looks for target cells to infect. Once again, the immune system attempts to stop the virus from entering cells by mounting an effective initial response, mainly with interferon. Natural killer cells increase in numbers and activity and go to work seeking out and killing viruses. The virus counters by releasing toxins that slow the immune response. The immune system can falter, but it rarely gives up.

While the battle rages, specialized components of the immune system promote the manufacture of memory cells against recurrent infection. The next time, the immune system will be prepared.

As the immune system gradually slows down viral replication, cytotoxic T-cells initiate the cleanup of remaining viruses. If all goes well, within a week or two, the body has returned to normal.

WHO'S MOST AT RISK?

If you have asthma or other chronic respiratory disorder, or a degenerative disease such as diabetes, you are more likely to catch the flu and suffer greater symptoms. Those with immune deficiency disorders are also more at risk. If you take immune-suppressing drugs such as cortisone, you will be more susceptible to infections.

People with hemochromatosis, a genetic condition that causes the accumulation of iron in tissues, are more easily infected because excess iron weakens immunity. Malnourishment and poor dietary choices lower immunity because there are not enough nutrients to supply the building blocks that make our immune systems strong.

The elderly are particularly vulnerable because of the lowered immunity that accompanies aging. Older people are less active and, if already ill or frail, spend most of their time in bed. Lying down facilitates accumulation of fluid in the lungs and increases the risk of pneumonia. During a typical garden-variety flu season, 90 percent of those killed by the flu are older people. It would be much the same during a flu pandemic.

Young children are also more susceptible because their immune systems are not yet experienced flu fighters. Mothers pass on some of their immunity to the fetus through the placenta and to infants in breast milk. Still, young children have a narrow range of immunity until they are exposed as they grow to a variety of pathogens. As we age, our antibody spectrum becomes increasingly broad. Like a library, the immune system keeps adding volumes and categorizing them in easy-access files.

BIRD FLU IMMUNE ALERT

Healthy adults and children with active immune systems have more aggressive disease progression and higher rates of death from the bird flu virus. The same pattern occurred during the Spanish flu of 1918; more young adults succumbed than other age groups. A similar pattern occurred among SARS victims. The problem lies in the immune system's response. As previously noted, when the immune system is overly aggressive, massive inflammation occurs in the lungs and can lead to suffocation.

A weak immune system will make you more vulnerable, but overly aggressive immunity can kill. Pandemic influenza strains are different from ordinary flu. Read the information in this chapter carefully. Don't try to overstimulate your immune system by taking more than the recommended dosage. Hyperactive immunity may be harmful to your health.

Beating the Flu

BUILD UP YOUR IMMUNITY

What you eat plays a role in viral immunity. Eating healthfully and getting proper nourishment promote a strong immune system. Don't overeat. It's bad for your health and weakens your immune system. Avoid extreme diets. The immune-powering diet is high in naturally occurring antioxidants, low in animal grease and margarines, high in vegetable and fish oils, and rich in fresh fruits and vegetables, and contains sufficient protein and moderate complex carbohydrates such as legumes and squashes. To keep your immune system vital, you need more fruits and vegetables than the recommended five to six servings a day. Eat eight to ten servings, preferably organic, every day.

Water is as important as food. Keep up your fluids and when you are sick, especially if you have a fever, drink at least eight to ten glasses of water daily. Don't drink tap water, unless it's boiled first; rather, use purified or natural spring water. Don't drink highly sugared carbonated beverages.

A healthy lifestyle supports viral immunity. Don't smoke or drink alcohol in excess. A few cocktails or glasses of wine on occasion are, however, actually good for your health. To maintain fitness and support immunity, exercise regularly. Don't overdo it! Intense exercise can temporarily reduce the population of important immune cells in the body.

To keep your viral immunity strong, don't get run down. Rest counters the effects of stress, relaxes the mind, promotes healing after illness, supports recovery after exercise, and improves immunity.

Getting enough deep sleep is vital for viral immunity. We are more susceptible to infection when deprived of sleep. Our immune chemistry is rebalanced during sleep. Protect yourself from infection by getting enough sleep. The average healthy night's slumber is between seven and nine hours. Some people can get away with less, others need more. Animals and children sleep more when they're sick. Take the tip. If you catch the flu, try the pillow prescription: Sleep between ten and 12 hours to speed recovery.

TEN WAYS TO ENHANCE YOUR IMMUNITY

1. EAT 8–10 SERVINGS OF FRUITS AND VEGETABLES.

2. CONSUME HEALTHFUL FATS AND OILS.

3. GET ENOUGH PROTEIN.

4. DON'T OVEREAT.

5. DRINK 8–10 GLASSES OF PURE WATER DAILY.

6. EXERCISE REGULARLY.

7. DON'T SMOKE.

8. DRINK ALCOHOL IN MODERATION.

9. REST WHEN TIRED.

10. GET ENOUGH SLEEP.

NATURAL IMMUNE MODULATORS

Immune modulators including milk products, mushroom extracts, and algae are substances that have regulating effects on the immune system. When commercially prepared to pharmaceutical standards, they are referred to as immunoceuticals.

Natural immune-modulating compounds tune up the immune system. They boost immunity by enhancing B-cell and T-cell function, increasing production of interferon, stimulating natural killer cell activity, and increasing the number of natural killer cells in circulation. Immune modulators also help manage the inflammation associated with infection. They are used to prevent viral infection, to help the immune system counter the virus and slow down the viral spread during infection, and to help the immune system clear remaining viruses from the body after infection. Many are also potent antioxidants that scavenge cellular debris left during and after infection.

GOT MILK? IMMUNE BOOSTERS IN MILK PRODUCTS

Whey protein contains many amino acids of high biological value necessary for health and longevity, as well as numerous immune-enhancing substances. Consuming 12 grams daily in the form of a protein shake helps strengthen immunity and can promote faster recovery from the flu. For people over 35, taking a pancreatic enzyme supplement with your protein shake helps it digest better. Adding 50 mg of vitamin B6 promotes protein synthesis in the body.

Though these products are made from milk, they are highly purified and contain only trace amounts of allergenic milk proteins and lactose. Even people who are allergic to dairy products or are lactose intolerant should be able to take these products. If you have a history of reacting to milk or suspect that you are highly sensitive to dairy products, however, start slowly with a fraction of the recommended amount and gradually increase it. If you notice any allergic symptoms, discontinue immediately.

Colostrum: The first pre-milk substance, colostrum, is produced by the mother's mammary glands in the few days just after giving birth. This "first" mother's milk contains immune-modulating substances to protect the newborn from infection. To accomplish this amazing immunological feat, nature comes well equipped. Colostrum is loaded with immunoglobulins, which promote the immune response, as well as other immune-boosting substances such as lactoferrin, transfer factors, fibronectin, enzymes, polypeptides (which boost T-cell numbers), a variety of cytokines, vitamins and minerals, and growth factors that promote healing.

Whole purified and concentrated colostrum that is commercially prepared from organically raised dairy cattle is an effective immune booster. Although it can destroy many common harmful gut bacteria and some viruses, it doesn't have direct activity against influenza. It's useful as a supportive nutritional supplement, however, and along with whey protein can bolster an aging immune system. It's safe and effective for children.

An average dosage of colostrum is 1–4 grams of powder or two to eight 450 mg capsules daily on an empty stomach. Not all bovine colostrum products are created equal. Choose a product that is cold processed, comes from pesticide- and hormone-free certified organic dairy cattle, and contains no less than 15% immunoglobulins. For greater protection, select a product that is standardized to contain 40% IgG, an important immunoglobulin that neutralizes toxins. Since products differ according to manufacturer, follow the label advice for brand-specific dosages.

Lactoferrin: An abundant protein component of colostrum, lactoferrin binds to iron in the body and makes it less available. Iron is necessary for life because it helps carry oxygen in the blood. When your body's iron supply is low, it can cause anemia. Iron is also used, however, by pathogenic microbes such as bacteria and viruses to promote their own growth. Since iron is recycled in the body, we don't need extra amounts other than what is provided in the diet or if we are anemic or losing blood as women do during menstruation. Lactoferrin's ability to regulate iron influences immune cells responsible for fighting infection. It is a safe product and recommended dosages range from 250 to 750 mg daily.

Transfer Factor: Immunological information is passed from mother to infant in the colostrum through the action of transfer factor. It trains the immune system. Transfer factor enhances natural killer cell activity, increases interferon production, and helps antigen recognition. It is safe to take, with recommended dosages ranging from 250 to 1,000 mg daily.

MUSHROOM POWER: IMMUNE-ENHANCING FUNGI

Mushrooms are well known for their immune-modulating properties. More than 50 different species have been researched with promising results in the treatment of cancer and for their effects against viruses. They are safe to take and are useful in rebuilding the immune system. The most efficient way to take them is in combinations that supply two or more immunoceutical mushroom extracts in one comprehensive formula. Sterile extracts for injection or intravenous use are available in Asia.

Ganoderma (Ganoderma lucidum): Called *reishi* in Japanese and *ling zhi* in Chinese, this mushroom is venerated in Asia as a longevity medicine. It has antiviral and immune-enhancing effects and is safe to take, with no known contraindications. Ganoderma is found in combination formulas with other mushrooms or Chinese herbs. The average dosage is 250–750 mg daily.

Maitake (Grifola frondosa): This Japanese healing treasure contains a unique beta-glucan, maitake D-fraction, which has been shown to have potent immune-enhancement and antitumor effects. It enhances the cell killing activity of macrophages; increases interleukin-1 production, which activates cytotoxic T lymphocytes; and promotes natural killer cell activity. Maitake D-fraction comes in a liquid extract form. The recommended dosage is 5–6 drops three times daily for health maintenance, and 15–20 drops three times daily for therapeutic purposes. It is safe and without side effects.

Shiitake (Lentinus edodes): Like all the medicinal mushrooms described in this section, shiitake's reputation as a healing substance is supported by a considerable amount of scientific research and has an excellent safety record. Shiitake's key ingredient is a polysaccharide called lentinan. The commercial preparation is called *Lentinus edodes* mycelium extract (LEM). Traditionally, shiitake is consumed fresh or dried, prepared in soups or vegetable dishes. The recommended dosage of LEM extract is 1–3 grams two to three times per day.

Cordyceps (Paecilomyces hepiali): Another highly prized traditional Chinese medicine for endurance and energy, and to improve lung function, Cordyceps sinensis is composed of the fungus cordyceps and the dried body of the larva of the moth on which it grows. Its active ingredients are polysaccharides, adenosine, and cordycepic acid. The immune-modulating and anti-inflammatory properties of cordyceps work by increasing levels of interferon, interleukin-1 and -2, regulating tumor necrosis factor, stimulating natural killer cell activity, and activating T helper cells. It is safe even in the high dosages necessary to improve viral immunity. The average dosage is 500–1,000 mg daily.

THE HEALTHY SEA: ANTIVIRAL ALGAE AND BACTERIA

Saltwater and freshwater algae have a long history as foods and medicines. The most important immune modulators among them are the blue-green algae. They stimulate immune-fighting cells that help prevent infection.

Spirulina (*Spirulina maxima*): A filamentous bacterium found in blue-green algae, spirulina influences the immune system by stimulating phagocytosis, the engulfing of diseased cells, and increasing interferon production, as well as activating T, B, and natural killer cells, thereby increasing the body's infection-fighting capabilities. Research has shown that, by preventing viruses from breaking through cell membranes, spirulina can protect against infection from many viruses including influenza A. The average dosage is four to six 500 mg tablets daily with a maximum dose of 5,000 mg daily. Spirulina also comes in a powdered form that can be mixed in water or juice. A specialized extract, Calcium-Spirulan (Ca-SP), isolated from *Spirulina platensis*, is composed of numerous sugars and calcium. According to the manufacturer, the additional calcium component is essential for its enhanced antiviral effect.

There is no toxicity associated with taking spirulina and it is considered safe to take during pregnancy; however, those with a metabolic condition called phenylketonuria (PKU) should discuss potential use of spirulina with their healthcare provider. This rare condition, characterized by an inability to metabolize the amino acid phenylalanine, could be aggravated by the rich mixture of amino acids found in spirulina.

9
The Food Factor

Kitchen Health to Beat the Flu

Foods not only nourish and sustain our bodies, but also are rich in compounds that prevent disease and fight infection. Fruits and vegetables such as oranges, papayas, apples, kale, carrots, and onions contain important vitamins and minerals that fortify the immune system. Many have antioxidant properties. Antioxidants are compounds that reverse the damaging effects of oxygen utilization by cells. Like a fire that needs air to burn, our cells require oxygen to produce energy and sustain life. But unlike a fire that burns out unless more fuel is added, our cells constantly regenerate themselves with the help of antioxidants. The flame of life cannot go out, yet must not consume itself. To keep the flame burning, choose fresh organic fruits and vegetables.

Avoid foods that destroy health and weaken immunity. These

immune-busting foods include refined sugar, processed foods, highly preserved and chemical laden packaged foods, and foods with pesticide and chemical fertilizer residue. Eating these foods undermines your natural immunity and inhibits healing and recovery.

Certain foods have properties that strengthen the immune system and some may even prevent the flu. Oats and mushrooms contain beta-glucan, an immune stimulant discussed in the last chapter. Yogurt contains friendly bacteria that help neutralize toxins in the gut, keep infectious bacteria and yeast under control, promote intestinal health, and support mucosal immunity critical to maintaining an effective barrier against invading viruses. Citrus fruits contain vitamin C that shortens the duration of a cold. The best flu-fighting foods are found in the vegetable section of your local supermarket or health food store and include garlic, ginger, green onions, chili peppers, and culinary herbs. Green tea is also beneficial.

In China, unlike in the West, foods are regarded as medicine. There are even restaurants that employ doctors specially trained in the medicinal value of foods. They diagnose the customer's complaint and prescribe an individualized menu composed of healing foods. Therefore the majority of foods discussed in this chapter are from the medicinal culinary art of Asia.

CHICKEN SOUP

Long considered one of nature's best remedies for a cold and the flu, chicken soup does a body good. But does it actually prevent or reduce the severity of upper respiratory tract infections and is it safe during a pandemic of avian virus? When tested by scientists, old-fashioned chicken soup was found to have anti-inflammatory effects. Drinking the warm broth helps hydrate the body and sooths a sore throat, and the steam clears nasal congestion. Herbs and vegetables cooked with the chicken offer the added advantage of supplying vitamins and minerals to help the immune system. It's unlikely that your doctor will send you home with a recipe for chicken noodle soup and a box of tissue instead of your flu shot. But is chicken soup helpful?

Stephen I. Rennard, M.D., chief of pulmonary medicine at the University of Nebraska Medical Center, thinks so. Dr. Rennard provided one piece of evidence why chicken soup, referred to as "Jewish penicillin," helps upper respiratory tract infections. He theorized that it might have effects on how our body's immune system responds to viral infections and then proceeded to test chicken soup in the laboratory. The target of his research was one of the main immune cells, the neutrophil. The most abundant type of white blood cells, neutrophils are responsible for activating

DR. WILLIAMS'S
CHICKEN SOUP + JALAPENOS

1–5 lb whole chicken

6 garlic cloves

1 medium-sized fresh ginger root

3 large red onions

12 large carrots

6 celery stalks

3 medium white or yellow potatoes

1 bunch parsley

1 bunch fresh oregano or 1 tsp dried oregano flakes

2 green or red jalapeno peppers

Clean chicken and put in a large pot of cold water. Bring to a boil. Add peeled and chopped garlic and ginger. Boil for 1/2 hour. Skim some of the fat off as it develops.

Add chopped onions, carrots, celery, and potatoes. Simmer for an additional 45 minutes.

Add parsley and oregano, and for greater tang, add chopped jalapeno peppers without the seeds. Cook another 15 minutes. Salt and pepper to taste. Serve.

phagocytes, cells capable of engulfing and destroying foreign objects and microorganisms. What Dr. Rennard speculated was that there is an unknown component in chicken soup that slows down neutrophil migration. Too many neutrophils in lung tissue produce excess inflammation that is exactly what causes much of the respiratory symptoms of the flu. Though more research is needed, these results demonstrate that chicken soup is indeed helpful when you have a cold or the flu.

Long before your grandmother was making chicken soup, the Chinese were cooking up their own version. For best results, according to Chinese tradition, use a black-skinned, all dark meat chicken with white feathers. Prized for its health properties, this unique breed of chicken is slowly cooked for hours along with ginger, garlic, rice, and ginseng root. The result is a nourishing tonic soup that fends off colds and beats the flu.

TRADITIONAL CHINESE CHICKEN AND RICE SOUP

1–3 lb chicken, clean and remove the skin

6 fresh garlic cloves

1 medium-sized fresh ginger root

1 cup sweet white or brown rice

8 slices of red ginseng root

Place the chicken in a slow cooker or deep baking pan. Add water to cover the chicken. Add peeled and chopped garlic and ginger. Cook or bake slowly for one hour. Add rice and sliced ginseng root. Cook until the chicken falls off the bone. Salt and pepper to taste.

Although chicken soup may be beneficial, would it be safe to consume during a bird flu pandemic? Even among chickens, avian influenza virus spreads by droplets of moisture coughed or sneezed into the air. It's a fatal disease in birds. Public health and veterinary experts contend that chicken meat or eggs are not dangerous to eat. Vertical transmission or infection passed on from a parent to offspring, they say, doesn't occur in chickens infected with bird flu. But given that emerging viruses are smart and SARS, another viral respiratory disease, spread via eating the meat from infected animals, it may be wise during a bird flu pandemic to avoid chicken soup and even eggs unless proven without a doubt to be safe. Instead, use vegetarian flu-fighters like umeboshi plums, kimchi, green onions, garlic, and ginger.

UMEBOSHI PLUMS

The word *umeboshi* in Japanese means "dried plum." In fact, these Asian delicacies are prepared by packing them in sea salt, so they are also called pickled plums.

Honored as a healing food in Korea and Japan, umeboshi plums were traditionally used to prevent fatigue, purify water, eliminate toxins in the body, and treat epidemic diseases. They are rich in organic acids that have an alkalinizing effect on the body. Maintaining alkaline versus acidic blood helps prevent disease and infection. Paradoxically, the high citric acid content in this pink-purple health food aids in breaking down unhealthy acids in the body, promotes the absorption of minerals, and neutralizes toxins—all of which promote healthful acid-alkaline balance, helpful in reducing inflammation during acute infection.

The pink color of the umeboshi plum comes from pickling the plums with the reddish-purple leaves of perilla (*Perilla frutescens*), a plant used in Asian cooking as a garnish and for its aromatic qualities. A Chinese variety is used as a tea to stop coughs and loosen up mucus during a cold. Research shows that perilla leaf contains natural substances that increase phagocytic activity, in which specialized cells devour microbes and diseased cells.

You can purchase umeboshi plums in Asian markets, health food stores, and macrobiotic stores. They come in small jars and should be kept refrigerated. Add one or two plums to soups, eat them as they come from the jar, or add one to your cup of green tea.

KIMCHI

A litany of praises regarding its health-enhancing qualities is attached to this strong-smelling Korean staple. Made with pickled vegetables, usually Chinese or Napa cabbage, with red chili peppers, onions, garlic, and anchovies, kimchi keeps cholesterol under control, promotes intestinal health, and helps to prevent diabetes. During the SARS epidemic, kimchi power is reported to have kept this deadly virus from spreading in Korea. Researchers in Seoul have even fed bird-flu-sickened chickens kimchi in an attempt to see if it could prevent infection or cure avian influenza. Though avian flu is usually fatal to chickens, more than half the kimchi-fed birds survived. It may be the strong acids in fermented foods along with the medicinal value of garlic, onions, and red chili with their bug-busting properties that make kimchi a star among foods that beat the flu.

Love it or loathe it, once you've tried it, you'll never forget the peppery taste and pungent smell of kimchi. You can buy it in Asian and health food stores. Use it like the Koreans do, as a side dish or garnish to spice up bland-tasting foods such as rice.

GARLIC AND ONIONS

If you think garlic (*Allium sativum*) is just for seasoning Italian cooking, think again. Research suggests that this humble member of the lily family can help lower cholesterol, reduce blood clotting, curb high blood pressure, and even prevent cancer. Garlic can also be a powerful treatment for infections. Like the onion, garlic contains allicin and other antibacterial compounds.

Also a member of the lily family, onions are rich in minerals and high in quercetin, a flavonoid with potent antioxidant activity. Quercetin also normalizes cytokines associated with immune reaction to infection.

The humble onion is like an undercover policeman. Used in

cooking, it can reduce inflammation, stop bacteria and parasites, lower cholesterol, prevent diabetes, and may reduce viral spread.

In particular, green onions or scallions have been used for centuries in China to prevent and treat the early stages of colds and flu. Add chopped scallions to soups or to garnish foods. Cook or steam whole scallions with fish or meats, or add flavor to the bland taste of tofu dishes. You can even make a tea with green onions. For flavor, add honey or an umeboshi plum.

GREEN TEA

Loaded with antioxidants and cancer-fighting properties, green tea polyphenols can block influenza virus from replicating. The medicinal effect of tea comes from catechins, a powerful class of antioxidant peculiar to green and white tea, principally epigallocatechin gallate (EGCG), which accounts for 50 percent of the total catechins in green tea leaves. When preparing green tea from tea bags, use at least two bags per cup for maximum effectiveness. When using the more traditional loose leaves, add one tablespoon of dried leaves per cup of hot water. Drink two cups of green tea daily.

FLU-FIGHTING CONDIMENTS, FLAVORINGS, AND SPICES

Tamari: Another potent alkalinizing Asian food is tamari, an aged and therefore stronger tasting version of soy sauce. It's a powerful antioxidant and also contains vitamins and minerals. Remember, tamari and soy sauce are high in sodium, so only use a little when flavoring foods.

Ginger: According to Asian culinary standards, no kitchen is complete without ginger and garlic. Ginger not only lends a spicy taste to foods, it helps balance the flavor of fish and other strong-tasting foods. The medicinal value of ginger is legendary. It treats digestive disorders, calms nausea, is a good remedy when women have menstrual problems, has anti-inflammatory effects, and promotes healthy circulation. Like garlic, ginger (*Zingiber officinale*) is touted for its ability to cure a variety of ailments, including reducing the symptoms of upper respiratory tract infections. Since influenza is a cold-weather illness, the warming properties of ginger help fortify the body against the flu.

You can buy fresh ginger in nearly any supermarket and all Asian food stores stock it. It can be added to chicken soup and other foods, but to treat the early symptoms of a cold or flu, ginger is best made into a tea. Peel the outer skin from a piece of fresh ginger root and slice it thinly or grate it to make two tablespoons. Steep in one cup of boiling water for ten minutes and add honey or lemon to taste. Drink warm for best results. To loosen chest congestion, make a poultice with dry powdered ginger.

To make a ginger poultice you'll need powdered dry ginger, water, and a 12x12 inch piece of linen or gauze. Mix 3 tablespoons of powdered ginger with a little warm water to form a paste. Microwave the paste for 30 seconds to heat it up and spread it on the linen or gauze so it covers completely about 1/8 inch thick. Apply the poultice, ginger side down, to the chest or upper back (over the lungs) and cover with a hot water bottle or electrical heating pad to maintain the heat. Leave it in place for at least 30 minutes. Some people have very sensitive skin, so if it burns take it off immediately to avoid irritation.

Red chili: Fiery foods are good for you. Cayenne pepper (*Capsicum frutescens*) and other varieties of chili peppers dilate the blood vessels, improve digestive function and intestinal tone, reduce pain, and have antibiotic properties. They temporarily speed up the body's metabolism, which can help you shed extra pounds. Red chili peppers contain twice the amount of vitamin C as citrus and have more beta-carotene than carrots.

Chili peppers stimulate the taste buds and perk up foods. Chop red chili peppers and add to soups or side dishes, or to garnish fish and other dishes. Dried chili powder, combined with parsley flakes or other dried culinary herbs, enhances the flavor of foods and has many of the same properties as fresh chilis. Mexican salsa made from fresh jalapenos, lime juice, cilantro, and salt is a south of the border staple.

Culinary spices: Many common kitchen herbs used to spice up foods and treat common ailments have flu-fighting properties.

DR. WILLIAMS'S FAMOUS "SALSA DE TRES CHILES"

8 Roma tomatoes, washed and diced

6 sprigs of cilantro, chopped

1/4 medium red onion

2 medium garlic cloves

1 green jalapeno and 1 red jalapeno

1 pastilla chili

Pinch of dried oregano

I've made this salsa countless times in Mexico, to the delight of my Latino guests. Place all the ingredients into a blender or food processor. Squeeze the juice from 5 limes and add one tablespoon of apple cider vinegar. Blend at medium speed. Salt to taste.

Culinary spices fight tumor necrosis factor, an immune chemical involved in acute inflammation and is released by white blood cells in response to infection. A little tumor necrosis factor is helpful in fighting infection, but too much causes massive inflammation and even tissue damage. Managing tumor necrosis factor production is important in your prescription to beat the flu. Green tea and curcumin (an ingredient in turmeric) are natural ways to control tumor necrosis factor.

Shikimic acid, found in Chinese star anise (Illicium verum), is actually the starting compound for making the antiviral drug Tamiflu. Spicing up your herbal teas with a few anise buds may not stop the flu, but it could be part of kitchen combat to keep your

FLU-FIGHTING CULINARY SPICES	
SPICE	**BENEFITS**
Anise (*Pimpinella anisum*)	Aids in digestion and helps stop coughing.
Basil (*Ocymum basilium*)	Helps clear head congestion during a cold.
Cardamom (*Elettaria cardamomum*)	Helps digestion of dairy products and soothes the stomach to treat indigestion.
Cilantro (*Coriandrum sativum*)	Helps prevent food poisoning and removes mercury from the body. Cilantro is the name of the young green leaves of the coriander plant.
Fennel (*Anethum foeniculum*)	Controls bad breath and, when chewed after spicy meals, masks the odor of garlic and onions.
Oregano (*Origanum vulgare*)	A favorite in Mediterranean cooking, oregano has powerful infection-fighting properties.
Peppermint (*Mentha piperita*)	Stops intestinal gas, calms indigestion, controls nausea, and sweetens the breath.

stomach calm and provide fluids when you're sick. Try a few drops of anise oil, like the French do in Provence, in a cup of hot water as a tea.

Turmeric or curry powder gives Indian food its yellow color and tanginess. It's also a well-known anti-inflammatory. Horseradish

FLU-FIGHTING CULINARY SPICES (CONTINUED)

SPICE	BENEFITS
Parsley (*Carum petroselinum*)	Promotes urinary flow and provides antioxidants.
Rosemary (*Rosmarinus officinalis*)	A powerful antioxidant, rosemary also has microbe-fighting properties, and it helps calm nerves.
Sage (*Salvia officinalis*)	Treats the congestion and stuffiness associate with colds, clears headaches, and kills parasites, bacteria, and yeasts. Sage oil may improve memory.
Thyme (*Thymus serpyllum*)	Wellknown as a natural antibiotic, it kills parasites and yeast. It can also soothe the chest and halt coughing.
Turmeric (*Curcuma domestica*)	The main ingredient in curry, turmeric adds zest and color to foods. It's cancer fighting and lowers unfavorable bacteria in the gut that cause gas and bloating. It has anti-inflammatory properties.

and mustard have properties that help clear sinus congestion and help you breathe better. Oregano has antimicrobial properties and, besides helping preserve and flavor Italian food, may actually help keep bacterial levels down in the body. For health benefits, use spices liberally in your cooking.

INFECTION-FIGHTING FOODS

FOOD	BENEFITS
Bananas	Soothe upset stomachs. Cooked green bananas stop diarrhea.
Bell Peppers	Loaded with vitamin C, green or red bell peppers are potent antioxidant foods.
Blueberries	Curb diarrhea, high in natural aspirin. Blueberry leaf tea may lower fevers and help with the aches and pains.
Carrots	Loaded with beta-carotene, raw carrots, and carrot juice increase the free-radical fighting capacity of your cells.
Chili Peppers	Loaded with vitamin A, chilis help open sinuses and break up mucus in the lungs.
Cranberries	Have properties that help prevent bacteria from sticking to cells lining the bladder and urinary tract.
Mustard & Horseradish	Help break up mucus in air passages.
Onions	Have phytochemicals that help the body clear bronchitis and other infections, and are rich in quercetin.
Orange Juice	Adds vitamin C and helps curb the flu.
Rice	Slows diarrhea.
Tea	Black and green tea contain catechin, a phytochemical purported to have natural antibiotic and anti-diarrhea effects.

FOOD AND DIETARY TIPS

✧ SHOP LOCALLY: THERE ARE HEALTH ADVANTAGES TO BUYING LOCALLY GROWN ORGANIC FOOD OVER COMMERCIALLY PROCESSED FOODS, BUT IN A PANDEMIC, SHOPPING FOR HOMEGROWN ITEMS MAY BE EVEN MORE IMPORTANT.

✧ SHOP ON THE OUTSIDE AISLES OF THE GROCERY STORE: THIS IS WHERE YOU FIND THE FRESH PRODUCE.

✧ BUY ORGANIC: CONSUMING FOODS FREE OF PESTICIDE RESIDUES AND CHEMICAL FERTILIZERS IS GOOD FOR YOUR HEALTH.

✧ STAY HYDRATED: DRINK PLENTY OF PURE WATER.

✧ EAT 8–10 SERVINGS OF FRESH FRUIT AND VEGETABLES DAILY.

✧ DRINK FRESH VEGETABLE JUICES SEVERAL TIMES A WEEK.

10
Natural Flu Solutions

How to Beat the Flu Using Natural Medicines

If you become infected with the influenza virus, one of the first things you need to do is reduce the viral burden on your body. The few antiviral medications we have are aimed at accomplishing this by destroying viruses or preventing their replication. Unfortunately, as already noted, they are not that effective, have unwanted side effects, have to be taken within the first 48 hours to be effective at all, and readily cause antiviral drug resistance.

Fortunately, nature has a remedy. The natural world provides an extraordinary array of antiviral substances in plants to deal with viruses without the disastrous side effects of drugs. One reason plants contain these antiviral compounds is that since they are rooted in the soil, they cannot run from danger as animals do and must make their own defenses. Plants have developed powerful biochemical arsenals to defend against insects, fungi, bacteria, and viruses.

Another reason why natural antiviral medications are important is because viruses find it difficult to become resistant to plant compounds. Unlike drugs, plant medicines don't exert immune pressures that stimulate the virus to mutate. Plants have complex molecules that work in concert with hundreds of other substances such as tannins, phenolic compounds, antioxidants, and trace minerals that inhibit viral replication and are less likely to cause antiviral resistance than drugs.

Our ancestors used plants to treat a wide range of diseases. In our times, scientists found that plants contain effective antiviral substances, confirming what our ancestors knew. Our bodies need these substances in plants to heal.

EVIDENCE-BASED NATURAL MEDICINE

Scientific evidence supports the use of natural medicine for immune boosting and virus fighting. Critics among medical doctors and skeptical scientists point to the lack of clinical trials that adhere to standards used for pharmaceutical drugs. However, this is not true. Though natural medicines have not been studied scientifically for as long as drugs, there is an overwhelming and growing body of evidence that natural medicines have therapeutic value.

The evidence-based model supports different levels of proof that a treatment works and is safe. The highest level, the gold standard for conventional clinical research, is the double-blind, placebo-controlled trial with enough subjects to arrive at statistically significant outcomes. The next level is review of a number of different studies using stringent criteria to see if there is a consensus among researchers about the effectiveness of a treatment.

Going down the ladder, but still of importance, are research studies that don't conform to the gold standard but are of clinical merit. The last level is expert opinion. In this type of evidence, an individual or a group of high professional standing approves of a therapy based on clinical data, even though it may not have the sanction of the highest levels of research. Following the evidenced-based model, all of the medications discussed in this chapter are supported by scientific and clinical evidence.

BEATING THE FLU NATURALLY

To beat a super flu, it is not only necessary to use effective and safe vaccines if they become available and antiviral drugs, as well as antibiotics for secondary bacterial infections, and to follow strict public health measures, it's also essential to employ natural immune boosters and antiviral medicines.

Natural antiviral medicines are biological substances that destroy viruses or prevent them from multiplying in your cells. They may be used alone, to complement other therapies, or as adjuncts to help drugs work better. They may also be valuable in the prevention and treatment of mild secondary infections, to expel congested mucus from the lungs, and to reduce inflammation in the body. As comfort measures, they can improve sleep, help relaxation, aid digestion, relieve constipation and diarrhea, and soothe sore muscles. During recovery, they can restore energy and help clean up the lymph system. There are many excellent books on herbal medicine, which I recommend you read for more information, but for the purpose of our discussion, let's concentrate on those that beat the flu.

Herbs make up the majority of antiviral substances. They come from a wide range of different plant families and from locations around the world. Some are gathered in the wild; others are grown commercially. Some of the most important ones are homeopathically prepared and others are only available as injections that have to be administered by a qualified healthcare practitioner. Many herbal antiviral medicines are prepared to pharmaceutical standards and come in concentrates and standardized extracts.

The natural antiviral medicines discussed in this chapter are divided into immune-boosting antiviral supplements, natural antibiotic, antiviral, and anti-inflammatory herbal medicines, antiviral homeopathic medicines, and traditional Chinese antiviral herbal medicines. Study the information on each medication carefully before use; if you have questions, consult a physician knowledgeable in the use of natural antiviral medicines.

HERBAL TEAS THAT BEAT THE FLU

✧ **Boneset:** Brew 2–3 tablespoons of dried boneset leaves and stems per cup of hot water. Simmer on the stove for 20 minutes. Keep covered while simmering. Add honey and drink 1 cup three times daily.

✧ **ELDERBERRY FLOWER:** Steep 2–3 tablespoons of dried elderberry flowers in boiled water for 10 minutes. Keep covered while steeping. Add honey and drink 1 cup three times daily.

✧ **GINGER:** Make a tea from 4–5 slices of fresh ginger per cup of hot water. Drink 1 cup three times daily.

✧ **SAGE:** Brew 2–3 tablespoons of dried sage leaves per cup of hot water. Simmer on the stove for 20 minutes. Keep covered while simmering. Add honey and drink 1 cup three times daily.

✧ **YARROW FLOWER:** Brew 2–3 tablespoons of dried yarrow flowers per cup of hot water. Simmer on the stove for 20 minutes. Keep covered while simmering. Add honey and drink 1 cup three times daily.

IMMUNE-BOOSTING ANTIVIRAL SUPPLEMENTS

Natural immune-boosting supplements are biological compounds that stimulate white blood cells to become more immunologically active thereby making them more successful against fighting infection. In chapter 8, I presented several of these compounds that help modify and regulate immunity without overly stimulating the immune system. In this section, I discuss one more important supplement useful in the fight against influenza.

Beta-glucan: Beta 1,3-D and 1,3/1,6 glucans are potent biological response modifiers with broad-spectrum antimicrobial activity against bacterial, fungal, parasitic, and viral infections. Beta-glucan has immune-modulating potential, antioxidant properties, and anti-tumor effects. It helps initiate a total rapid immune response without overly stimulating the immune system and doesn't induce antibody production against itself. This is an advantage when treating infection because overactive defenses can cause more damage than the virus.

The scientific evidence for beta-glucan is very favorable. It has been used to treat influenza A and B, human herpesvirus and other viruses, and even destroys anthrax. Beta-glucan appears to work by stimulating macrophages (microbe-digesting cells that are part of the first-line defense response) and natural killer cells. These important virus-fighting cells have receptors that exhibit a specific affinity for beta-glucan. When stimulated, macrophages inhibit viral replication, slowing down the spread of infection in the body. Beta-glucan also increases cytotoxic cells that help clean up viruses and tissue debris after infection.

Beta-glucan not only increases disease resistance, but assists in wound healing and repair of cells. This could make a critical difference in the protection and recovery of damaged lung tissue caused by influenza infection. Beta-glucan can also serve as an adjuvant to improve the immunological action of vaccination.

The most common commercial form of beta-glucan is a pure isolated polysaccharide compound derived from baker's yeast (*Saccharomyces cerevisiae*), but beta-glucan is also found in oats, barley, and edible mushrooms, with portobellos having the highest content. Beta-glucan is considered safe and nontoxic. Not only does it have no known drug interactions, it may also help antibiotics work better. Even though it is derived from yeast, since it is a pure compound there are no reported allergic reactions among users with yeast or mold sensitivities. If you have yeast or mold allergies, however, talk with your doctor before using beta-glucan products.

Among the many beta-glucan products on the market, a Norwegian standardized 1,3/1,6 glucan used in research studies is considered to be 200 times more potent than echinacea as an immune booster and is favored by many doctors. Select a product that contains at least 60% beta 1,3/1,6 glucan and low fat, protein, and ash content. A typical oral dosage ranges from 100 mg to 500 mg daily for prevention, upward to 1,500 mg daily for the treatment of the common cold, and as high as 20,000 mg daily during an active infection.

VITAMINS AND MINERALS TO HELP BEAT THE FLU

In order to have strong viral immunity, it's necessary to eat a healthful diet with an abundance of fresh fruits and vegetables. Fresh, and preferably organic, produce contains nutrients essential for health and the prevention of disease. Another reason a diet rich in nutrients is important is that, when the influenza virus attacks the lungs, tissues suffer from a great deal of oxidative stress. Consuming supplemental antioxidants such as vitamins A, C, and E and the minerals zinc and selenium combat tissue damage. Of the many vitamins, minerals, and other nutrients found in foods, the following ones stand out as flu fighters.

Vitamin A: An essential for proper immune function, vitamin A helps maintain the tissue that makes up skin and mucous membranes. It's the mucous lining of the respiratory tract that serve as the first line of defense against viruses by preventing invading viruses from lodging on the surface of the lungs, throat, and nasal passages. Getting enough vitamin A helps keep the mucosal barrier strong against infection.

Vitamin A supplementation enhances the body's immune response to infection. Not enough vitamin A in the body makes us more vulnerable to viral infection. Mainly found in liver, eggs, fish, and milk, you can also get vitamin A by eating green leafy and brightly colored fruits and vegetables. They contain beta-carotene, which is converted in the body into vitamin A.

Though vitamin A is considered safe to take, too much can lead to toxic symptoms including nausea, vomiting, headache, and blurred vision. Chronically high amounts can cause birth defects, liver damage, and osteoporosis. For balanced dietary supplementation, take 15,000 IU of mixed carotenoids and 10,000 IU of vitamin A from fish oil daily with meals. A comprehensive high-potency multiple vitamin and mineral supplement usually contains these amounts. To upgrade your immune system, however, you'll need 20,000 IU or more daily. Since vitamin A can impair liver function, when taking higher dosages, use an aqueous or water-soluble form. For the treatment of respiratory tract infection and to help promote tissue healing, you'll need 80,000 IU daily. Don't take this amount for longer than three weeks. High dosages of vitamin A are best supervised by a physician.

Vitamin C: Although vitamin C has been extensively studied for its use in a variety of diseases including viral infection, there is limited data showing it to be clearly effective. Case studies in the medical and lay literature, however, and an overwhelming number of anecdotal reports testify to the fact that there's something miraculous about vitamin C therapy.

The elderly are particularly at risk for contracting the flu and suffering from severe postinfection consequences. Though the governmental policy is that all seniors should get a flu shot, it's estimated that influenza vaccination is only 30-40 percent effective in frail elderly people. Supplementing our seniors with a combination of vitamins C and E provides superior protection against the influenza, even with a flu shot.

The bottom line for vitamin C is that it's unlikely to do you any harm and can at least help to shorten the duration of sickness by a few days and speed recovery. Megadosing with vitamin C seems to offer the greatest protection. But how much is enough? Taking ascorbic acid crystals dissolved in water is the least expensive form, but it can be overly acidic for the digestive system of many people. An alternative is taking an effervescent powder buffered with calcium and magnesium. Capsules are also available. To treat the flu, take 1,000 mg every hour for the first 6–12 hours, then reduce to

1,000 mg three times daily. If you start to have abdominal bloating or diarrhea, reduce the dosage until symptoms are relieved. For daily protection, take 500 mg two to four times daily.

Since too much vitamin C causes diarrhea, very high dosages of vitamin C can only be administered intravenously by a physician. The reported lowest effective dosage for intravenously administered vitamin C is 30,000 mg with an upper limit of 100,000 mg.

Though vitamin C is safe and nontoxic, there are concerns about its long-term use. Patients on dialysis and those with chronic kidney disease, hemochromatosis (an iron-overload condition), gout, or kidney stones should avoid taking megadoses of vitamin C.

Vitamin E: The death rate from influenza among the elderly tends to be high. The cause is mainly due to pneumonia and secondary bacterial complications. Oxidative damage in the lungs is rampant during influenza infection. Vitamin E is highly protective against this kind of tissue damage. It also bolsters immune function. Supplementing with vitamin E can help reduce the risk of postviral infection. Take 1,000 IU of mixed tocopherols containing a minimum of 500 mg of d-alpha tocopherol. In these dosages, vitamin E is considered safe and without adverse interactions. Since it can interfere with platelet aggregation, however, do not take it if you take blood-thinning drugs such as coumadin or aspirin.

Selenium and zinc: These important antioxidant minerals are necessary for immune function. For daily supplementation during flu season, take 400 mcg of selenium and 30 mg of zinc. To treat influenza infection, you may need more, but both can be toxic in high dosages. Don't take more than the recommended amount without the supervision of a qualified healthcare provider.

Rhinoviruses, those that cause the common cold, don't fare well when exposed to zinc. Sucking on lozenges composed of zinc gluconate or acetate every few hours helps stop a cold and slow down the flu. They are safe for adults and the elderly, but should be used with caution for children so that they don't take too many and overdose. Zinc nasal sprays have not been proven effective. Clinical trials support the use of zinc lozenges to shorten the duration and symptoms of upper respiratory tract infections, but for the lozenges to be most effective, you need to start sucking on them within 24 hours after the first symptoms appear.

N-acetyl-L-cysteine (NAC): An amino acid derived from L-cysteine, a protein found in foods, NAC is a powerful antioxidant with affinity for lung tissue. NAC supports immune function and helps thin mucus, reduce inflammation, detoxify the liver, and protect against acetaminophen poisoning. It has a protective effect on the lungs during viral infections and can help increase the chance of surviving influenza. It is a safe substance but on rare occasions can cause dry mouth, dizziness, abdominal discomfort, and nausea. As with all nutrients, discuss any potential drug interactions with your doctor or pharmacist before taking them. The average dosage is 500 mg three times daily away from food.

Quercetin: This potent bioflavonoid is found in apple skins, red wine, red onions, tea, and raspberries. It has anti-inflammatory properties, is a natural antihistamine, has anti-cancer effects, has cardiovascular protective effects, inhibits viruses, and can improve respiratory function by reducing inflammation in the lungs. Its anti-inflammatory effects are due to its inhibition of interleukin-6 production and nuclear factor kappa-B, both inflammatory cytokines; and its inhibition of nitric oxide, a substance associated with inflammation. Quercetin also regulates the immune system's ability to normalize inflammation. It helps inflamed tissues recover faster and is useful in colitis. It is a safe substance without side effects. Take two to three 250 mg capsules twice daily.

NATURAL ANTIBIOTICS

Bacterial infection and massive inflammation are the two most common causes of mortality associated with influenza infection. To beat pandemic flu, it's not only necessary to increase resistance and fight the virus, it's important to control secondary bacterial infections that cause pneumonia. In this section, I discuss natural alternatives to antibiotics.

Grapefruit seed extract: Also known as citrus seed extract, this substance is processed from the seeds of grapefruit (*Citrus paradise)*. It has powerful antiseptic properties against antibiotic-resistant germs. Its broad-spectrum antimicrobial activity fights against bacteria, fungi, and viruses. It's commercially available in liquid concentrate or as a dry extract. Take two to five drops in six ounces of water or juice three times daily. The recommended dosage for the dry extract is 250 mg three times daily to treat an active respiratory tract infection. It is considered safe to use, but the liquid can irritate the skin and mucous membranes of the mouth and stomach, so when using the liquid concentrate always dilute it in water or juice.

Garlic (*Allium sativa*) extract: Concentrated garlic extracts containing the active ingredient allicin are useful in managing secondary bacterial infections of the upper respiratory tract. In my clinical experience, to treat infections with garlic, the more concentrated the better. Use a standardized extract containing at least 300 ppm pure allicin, which is the equivalent of 40 fresh garlic bulbs. One capsule twice daily is the average dose. To treat an active infection, you'll need to up the dose. Take two or three capsules three times daily.

Garlic is safe to take, even for prolonged use. Eventually, you'll exude the typical garlic odor, however. Odorless forms also have therapeutic benefit. For some people, concentrated garlic extracts cause nausea and abdominal discomfort due to gas. Use garlic extract in a concentration of 100:1 containing a minimum of 5.3 mg of scordinin, another highly prized garlic constituent. Take one 250 mg capsule twice daily with food. Increase the dose if necessary to treat severe infection. Combining garlic extracts with other flu-fighting herbs such as elderberry may provide added benefits over a single herb.

Myrrh (*Commiphora myrrha*): Known for its healing properties, myrrh is a resin from a tree and has a long history as a medicine in the Middle East and Asia; the resin was also burned at Roman funerals to mask the smell of the dead. Myrrh contains volatile oils and other compounds that have antimicrobial properties. It makes a very effective mouthwash and tooth gargle, helping relieve sore throat and kill germs lodged in the mucous membranes. To make a mouthwash, start with the alcohol tincture of myrrh and mix ten drops in four ounces of warm water.

Propolis: Another useful natural antiseptic, propolis is a resin collected by honeybees to keep the hive free from germs. The tincture makes an effective mouthwash and can be mixed with myrrh (see herbal medicines) or used by itself to treat sore throat. Mix one-third teaspoon of propolis tincture in one cup of warm water and gargle three times daily.

ANTIVIRAL AND ANTI-INFLAMMATORY HERBAL MEDICINES

In this section, I discuss herbs that treat viral infection and lower inflammation. In plants, nature has created its own combination therapy in the form of synergistic activity between therapeutic compounds. For example, antiviral herbs may have compounds with anti-inflammatory properties or immune-modulating activity. Therapeutic synergism enhances the effects of treatment and promotes healing.

Cat's Claw (*Uncaria tomentosa*): Cat's claw is widely used in the treatment of arthritis and other inflammatory diseases. It's also an immune-boosting medicine and has broad-spectrum antiviral activity. This is a safe herb without known adverse effects. It can, however, inhibit an important detoxification enzyme in the liver, making drugs stay in the body longer, which is not a benefit when you are taking a potentially toxic pharmaceutical drug at the same time as the cat's claw. As with most herbs, cat's claw shouldn't be taken by pregnant women.

The medicinal parts come from the inner bark and roots of an Amazonian vine. The recommended form is standardized to contain 3% oxindole alkaloids and 15% polyphenols. For the treatment of viral infections, take two 500 mg capsules of the standardized extract three times daily with food. Tinctures are also useful. Mix one-third tablespoon in a glass of water and take three times daily away from food.

Echinacea (*Echinacea purpurea, E. angustifolia, E. palida*): This low-growing wildflower native to the American West is extremely popular in Europe, where it is extensively cultivated and manufactured into cold and flu remedies. It is antiseptic, immune modulating, and anti-inflammatory, and has antibacterial and antiviral properties. The active immune-stimulating ingredients in echinacea are polysaccharides and the polyphenolic compound echinacosides, a caffeic acid derivative used as a biochemical marker for standardization.

At least 15 randomized, double-blind, placebo-controlled studies (the "gold standard" of medical research) suggest that echinacea may play a role in shortening the duration of upper respiratory tract infections caused by the common cold or flu. It appears to work by stimulating phagocytosis and increasing the number of white blood cells, creating a short-lived immune stimulation.

Echinacea is a safe herb without major side effects. It may be used during pregnancy and is safe for long-term use of several months or more. Minor side effects, including upset stomach, nausea, and dizziness, have been reported. Serious side effects include worsening of asthma symptoms and rare allergic reactions such as rash, swelling, and difficulty breathing in people with allergies to daisies, ragweed, marigolds, chrysanthemums, or related plants. Talk to your doctor right away if you experience side effects. In liquid form, it can cause a temporary mild tingling sensation of the tongue. Injectable forms can cause a mild, transient fever. Since it has immune-enhancing actions, echinacea should not be taken long term in progressive conditions involving increased autoimmunity such as rheumatoid arthritis.

The active compounds found in echinacea aren't easily extracted in water, making tea from the dried root useless. Tincture or liquid extracts made from the fresh whole plant are best. For the treatment of an active infection, take 1 teaspoon (about 300 mg) diluted in two ounces of water or juice, four times daily. Dry extracts are also effective, but there is concern that some of the products standardized to echinacoside phenols may not have enough polysaccharides, the other immune-stimulating compound found in echinacea. For best results, choose standardized extracts containing at least 4% echinacosides and 5% polysaccharides and take 400–1,200 mg daily, more if you have an acute infection. Select products guaranteed free of heavy metals and other contaminants. Injectable forms are also available.

BROAD-SPECTRUM ANTI-INFLUENZA HERBAL REMEDIES

These two herbs have a wide range of antiviral activity against influenza and other viruses. They are useful in treating mild symptoms of the flu and are best taken at the first onset of symptoms.

Elderberry *(Sambucus nigra)*: Effective against different influenza strains, elderberry contains novel type 2 ribosome-inactivating protein, a substance that has an inhibiting effect on viruses. The flowers are the medicinal part. To make a tea, steep 3–5 g of the dried flowers in one cup of boiled water for 10–15 minutes. Add honey and drink one cup three times daily. Elderberry is also available as a standardized extract. Choose one that contains 28% anthocyanins and take two 700 mg capsules three times daily when you have the flu.

Olive leaf extract *(Olea curopaea)*: Made from the leaves of the Mediterranean olive tree, olive leaf extract is used as a broad-spectrum antiviral. It is a safe medication with no known adverse effects or interactions. Use the standardized extract containing 17 to 23 percent oleuropein, one of the active components in the leaf. The average recommended dose is two 500 mg capsules twice daily.

ANTIVIRAL HOMEOPATHIC MEDICINES

The homeopathic Materia Medica (the Latin medical term for a body of therapeutic knowledge about substances used for healing) is filled with dozens of remedies for the treatment of flu-like symptoms. These include Eupatorium, prepared from the herb boneset, used to treat chills and fever accompanied by deep aching pains; Gelsenium, used when flu symptoms are accompanied by fatigue and body aches that come on gradually; and Aconite, used when symptoms come on suddenly.

These and other classical homeopathic remedies for the flu are well described by others. For the purposes of this book, I focus on modern homeopathically prepared medicines.

Beating the Flu

Oscillococcinum: This modern homeopathic remedy is specifically for influenza. Prepared from duck livers by the French homeopathic company Boiron, it has been shown to reduce the symptoms and duration of the flu. Like all medicines to treat the flu, it is important to begin taking Oscillococcinum at the first signs of symptoms. Take one dose of three pellets followed by one or two additional doses 6 and 12 hours later. There are no side effects with this medication and no conflicts with other drugs.

Echinacea compositum S: This medication is manufactured by Heel Biotherapeutics and is packaged in oral vials. It contains *Echinacea angustifolia* D3 and other homeopathic substances. It is useful to treat influenza and minor bacterial respiratory tract infections. The dosage is one oral vial under the tongue three times daily for acute conditions and one vial daily for ten days for chronic conditions. In Europe, it's available as an injection.

Engystol N: Another Heel product, this medication is useful for all acute and chronic viral diseases including influenza. It contains *Vincetoxicum* (swallow wort) and other homeopathic medicines and is used as supportive therapy for the flu. Dissolve one tablet in the mouth three times daily away from food, or more frequently for acute infection. It also comes in an injectable form that is available by prescription and administered by a licensed healthcare practitioner. One ampule is injected intramuscularly three times a week.

Gripp-Heel: Also from Heel, this medication contains *Eupatorium perfoliatum* (boneset) D3 and other homeopathic substances. It can be used alone or with herbs and other natural immune-boosting medicines to beat the flu. Dissolve one tablet in the mouth three times daily away from food and more frequently (once every 15 minutes) for acute infection. It is also available in injectable form.

TRADITIONAL CHINESE ANTIVIRAL HERBAL MEDICINES

Traditional Chinese medicine (TCM) and its modern adaptations cover all aspects of immune enhancement, influenza protection, and treatment for *ganmao*, seasonal flu, and *wen bing*, epidemic influenza. According to TCM, there are two equally important aspects to preventing and treating the flu. *Fu zheng,* the method of supporting vitality and immunity, is the first aspect. It involves fortifying the body by strengthening the constitution and enhancing immunity. The other is called *qu xie,* which implies clearing pathogenic influences from the body and involves taking antiviral, anti-inflammatory, and antifebrile herbal medicines. These two methods complement each other in overcoming illness and benefiting health.

There is good evidence that Chinese herbal medicine protects against viral infection by enhancing immunity, managing inflammation, and inhibiting viral replication. As discussed in chapter 7, during the SARS epidemic they may have been as useful as Western drugs and when used concurrently with drugs improved the effectiveness of treatment. Chinese medicine can also play a role during convalescence by nourishing the body so it recovers faster.

Many Chinese herbs, such as ginseng and astragalus, have powerful immune-modulating effects. They stimulate the production of interferons, inhibit viruses, and have anti-inflammatory effects, as well as virus-fighting properties. Others like andrographis and isatis are effective in the treatment of colds and flu.

INDIVIDUAL ANTIVIRAL CHINESE HERBS

Andrographis (*Andrographis paniculata*): *Chuan xin lian*/herba andrographis contains a group of compounds, andrographolides, useful in the treatment of common viral and bacterial infections. It's a safe herb, though traditional Chinese herbalists don't recommend taking it for longer than one to two weeks at a time. Commercially available in a preparation made in Europe, it's the best-selling cold and flu remedy in Scandinavia. Take one 300 mg tablet four times daily of the standardized extract containing 4% andrographolides; for severe infections, increase the dosage to two tablets four times daily.

Astragalus (*Astragalus membranaceus*): *Huang qi*/radix astragali is an adaptogenic tonic that helps restore the body's energy. Though it doesn't have direct antiviral activity, it has powerful immune-stimulating properties that raise interferon levels, one of the most important immune chemicals for fighting against viral invasion. Since it's a very safe herb, it can be taken over a long period of time. Astragalus can be made into a tea and used as a daily beverage for all ages. Simmer 9–30 g of the dried sliced root per two cups of water for 20 minutes. Let the decoction sit for another ten minutes and then drink warm. The dosage for encapsulated forms is two 500 mg capsules twice daily.

Bupleurum (*Bupleurum falcatum*): *Chai hu*/radix bupleuri contains groups of chemical compounds, saikosaponins and saikosides, which have antiviral, immune-stimulating, and anti-inflammatory actions. In TCM, bupleurum is used to treat unresolved respiratory tract infections. It's rarely used alone but combined with other herbs in the classic formula Minor Bupleurum Decoction. Bupleurum is considered a safe, nontoxic herb; however, it is traditionally recommended not to take it for longer than a few months. Drug interactions have occurred when it is taken concurrently with interferon.

Ginseng (*Panax ginseng*): *Ren shen*/radix ginseng is the king of Chinese herbal tonics. In addition to its adaptogenic properties, recent research has shown it to contain chemicals, polysaccharides, which have anti-inflammatory and antiviral properties. There are many forms of ginseng, but the best one for preventing, shortening the duration of, and recovering from the flu is North American ginseng (*Panax quinquefolium*). The standardized extract containing 80 percent polyfuranosyl-pyranosyl-saccharides is the preferred form and is manufactured in Canada. For prevention, take one 200 mg capsule twice daily during the flu season.

North American ginseng is considered a safe, nontoxic herb and can be taken by adults for several months without adverse effects. Korean or Chinese red ginseng can be use to strengthen the body and as a preventative during flu season, especially for the weak and elderly. It should not, however, be taken during high fever or by children.

Isatis (*Isatis tinctoria*): *Ban lan gen*/radix isatidis treats viral and bacterial infections and reduces inflammation. It can be combined with andrographis and other antiviral foods and herbs to make a potent antiviral herbal cocktail. One traditional Chinese infection-fighting combination includes isatis and andrographis along with dandelion (*Taraxacum mongolicum*) leaves and flowers. Prepared in a combination with other infection-fighting herbs, it also comes in granule form called *ban lan gen chong ji*. To make a tea, dissolve one packet in hot water and drink one cup three times daily.

Though considered a safe herb, isatis has been associated with allergic reactions. The average dosage for tea is 10–15 g of the dried root decocted for 30 minutes. Drink one cup three times daily. It also comes in tablets. Look for a 15:1 concentrated extract of the root and take 200 mg three times daily.

A leaf from the same indigo plant family, *da qing ye*/folium isatidis, is also useful, especially in the early stages of upper respiratory tract infections. It has anti-inflammatory properties, lowers fever, and exerts effects against bacteria and fungi. In China, it's used to treat the common cold and the flu.

Licorice (*Glycyrrhiza glabra*): One of the oldest herbal remedies in the world, *gan cao*/radix glycyrrhizae is anti-inflammatory and can inhibit viral replication. The active compound, glycyrrhizin, is contained in the root and was shown in the laboratory to outperform dramatically the antiviral drug ribavirin against the SARS virus. The effective dosage, however, is rather high, 4,000 mg, and has to be taken for many weeks. At that level, licorice can cause significant adverse effects if taken longer than one week. These include high blood pressure, swelling, hormone disruption, and fatigue.

In China, glycyrrhizin extract is available in concentrated oral forms as well as administered by intramuscular injection or intravenously. Injectable forms are not approved as drugs in the United States.

This medication could prove valuable during a bird flu pandemic and deserves further scientific investigation. Because of the possibility of serious side effects, only use licorice extracts under the supervision of a knowledgeable licensed healthcare practitioner.

CHINESE ANTIVIRAL FORMULAS

For centuries, Chinese herbal pharmacies have been preparing patented preparations as pills and liquid extracts. In modern times, classical formulas for the treatment of respiratory tract infections are also made in fast-dissolving extracts packaged in individual foil packets. Though these formulas have similar ingredients, each has slightly different clinical applications. Consult a specialist in traditional Chinese herbs for details. They are found in Asian markets and Chinese herb shops, and can also be obtained from your local acupuncturist.

Gan Mao Ling: This modern anti-influenza combination contains isatis and Chinese honeysuckle flowers (*flos lonicera*), along with other infection-fighting herbs. It comes in pills and instant granules for making into tea. The dosage of the pill form is five tablets three times daily. If using the granule form, *gan mao tui re chun ji*, dissolve one packet in one cup of hot water and drink one cup three times daily.

Ge Xian Weng: This preparation contains extracts of isatis leaf and root, dandelion flower and leaf, and *zi hua di ding*/herba violae (*Viola yedoensis*), another infection-fighting plant from the Chinese antiviral arsenal. For the treatment of the flu, dissolve one packet into one cup of hot water. The dosage is one cup three times daily away from food.

Yin Qiao San: Widely used remedy in China for the treatment of febrile disease, this formula is best used in the early stages of the flu when there is fever. The principal herbs are *jin yin hua*/flos lonicerae (*Lonicera japonica*) and *lian qiao*/fructus forsythiae (*Forsythia suspense*). Used together, they have synergistic activity against influenza. The dosage is two to three tablets three times a day or more frequently for acute symptoms.

Zhong Gan Ling: Known as "serious effective cold and flu tablets," this formula is best used when headache and sore, swollen throat accompany the flu. The recommended dosage is five tablets three times daily.

INDIVIDUALIZED CHINESE HERBAL FORMULAS

Traditionally, Chinese herbal medicines are a personalized prescription to meet the individual needs of each patient. After an extensive examination and history taking, the doctor of Chinese medicine prepares the formula that addresses each aspect of the patient's condition. The prescription for the treatment of influenza in older people, for example, will contain antiviral herbs along with tonics such as ginseng to restore vitality. Herbs that help the expectoration of mucus or quell fever may also be added. Most large cities have traditional Chinese herbalists and clinics where you can receive treatment with Chinese herbs.

11
Maximize Your Strategy to Beat the Flu

Doctor-Assisted Solutions

Up till now, this book has provided you with self-directed strategies for the prevention and treatment of influenza. This information is meant to help you improve your chances of survival and aid in restoring health after infection. Should you become seriously ill with pandemic influenza, however, the preferred method of administering medications is by intramuscular injection and intravenous therapies, or directly to the mucous lining of the nasal or respiratory passage by sprays or in a nebulizer. Drawing on my 25 years of clinical experience from treating influenza and other viral infections, these doctor-assisted solutions are, in my professional opinion, among the best ways to maximize your chances of beating pandemic influenza.

Beating the Flu

Finding the right doctor is crucial to effective and safe treatment. Unless you have a referral from a trusted source, approach your medical care, including natural solutions, as you would any other important life decision: Be adequately prepared, well informed, and cautious. Be responsible by studying the material in this chapter carefully before approaching your doctor.

I recommend that you seek a holistic medical doctor (M.D.), osteopathic doctor (D.O.), naturopathic doctor (N.D. or N.M.D.), or doctor of Oriental medicine (D.O.M. or O.M.D.) who is amenable to administering these therapies should you or a family member require them. Inquire if they use any of the treatments covered in this chapter. You may want to show them a copy of this book. Some physicians may not be receptive to your inquiry, others will be curious, and still others may already use these medications or provide you with a referral to a colleague who does.

Should a pandemic threat become real, make contact with your doctor immediately. Don't wait until you're deathly ill to request treatment. If you have stockpiled any of these medications, make arrangements with your doctor to administer them for you in a timely manner.

OPENING NATURE'S MEDICINE CHEST: BIOLOGICAL IMMUNOTHERAPIES

Immunotherapy describes a group of different treatments utilizing biological elements to stimulate functions of the body's own natural defense system. Immunotherapeutic agents are also referred to as biological response modifiers. When it's a question of prevention and healing, biological therapies, as opposed to chemical therapies, rely on the body's own mechanisms and systems instead of inducing toxic responses.

The goal of biological immunotherapies is to protect the body from developing diseases and to help with recovery if a disease arises. Here are some biological immunotherapies that have the potential to boost the immune system for prevention of and as an aid in recovery from the flu. All of these therapies must be administered by a qualified physician.

Intravenous immunoglobulin (IVIg): This therapy involves the infusion of immunoglobulins into a vein by slow drip. Immunoglobulins are disease-fighting proteins called antibodies, which are found in human blood and ward off harmful bacteria, viruses, and other germs. IVIg is biologically similar to gamma globulin, a natural product manufactured from human serum, administered by intramuscular injection, and used since the 1950s to prevent hepatitis infection by giving the body a temporary immune boost. Theoretically, immunoglobulins should also work against influenza virus.

Extensive use over a period of years has demonstrated that IVIg is a safe, nontoxic therapy with virtually no side effects. Intramuscular injections of gamma globulin are considered safe and are screened to be free of impurities and contagious viruses. IVIg or intramuscular injections of gamma globulin may interact with live virus vaccines, reducing their immunization effectiveness. Since immunoglobulins are proteins, even purified medical forms may cause allergic reactions.

Interferon: One of the first lines of defense against viral infection, the body's own interferon serves as an effective flu fighter. The H5N1 bird flu strain, however, has found ways to dodge interferon defense mechanisms in the body. It's possible that giving interferon could stimulate the body's own interferon defenses or directly inhibit the virus. Low-dose interferon nasal or throat sprays have been used to shorten the duration of symptoms. High-dose interferon, as is used to treat hepatitis C, is associated with significant adverse reactions including extreme weakness, severe headache, and muscle aches. Low-dose interferon, however, when administered for a short period of time, is considered to be free of side effects and could prove effective in enhancing viral immunity.

Homeopathic interferon is another option. The value of the homeopathic preparation is that it may serve as an immune regulator rather than overstimulate defenses, an important issue when excess cytokine production is responsible for many of the symptoms associated with bird flu. Injectable homeopathic interferon is available in Europe.

Beating the Flu

When small amounts of low-dose interferon are injected into acupuncture points in a technique called biopuncture, the entire body becomes attenuated with immune-regulating medication. This provides a global healing effect without overly stressing the body with large single doses of medication. This technique is used in China with all injectable medications discussed in this chapter, as well as antibiotics and steroids. The principle behind the practice of acupuncture point injection is that smaller amounts of a medication if given at the right time and in specific sites on the body have a greater synergistic effect with fewer adverse reactions then larger dosages.

Thymus extract: Whole thymus glandular extracts from animals have been in use for decades. Most are made from organic bovine sources and are processed into tablets or capsules. Injectable forms are also available; in my clinical experience, these are more effective than pills. Thymodulin is an approved drug in Italy and exported worldwide except to the United States. Thymu-Uvocal and other thymus extracts for injection are available in Germany. Synthetic thymosin is available by prescription in the United States.

Injected thymus extract has been shown to be helpful in reducing the frequency of viral respiratory tract infections. It energizes the immune system. As an influenza vaccine adjuvant, synthetic thymosin improves immunization rates in older people. Thymus extract is considered safe and without toxic effects. As with all medicinal protein substances, allergic reactions are possible but extremely rare.

DHEA: Dehydroepiandrosterone (DHEA) is an androgenic (a substance associated with male features) hormone with immune enhancing properties. Levels fall during aging, and supplementation with DHEA, especially for the elderly, can help improve resistance to infection. Scientific studies have shown that taking DHEA boosts immunity in aging subjects and it may enhance the effect of influenza immunization. Although available as an oral nutritional supplement in health food stores, it is best to have your physician test your blood levels before starting a course of supplementation. DHEA is generally considered safe, but in some people when taken in higher than recommended dosages it can cause high blood pressure, acne, and anxiety. The average dosage is between 25 and 100 mg daily taken with food. DHEA may work even better if taken with vitamin D as found in cod liver oil. It can also be applied to the skin as a cream.

INTRANASAL MISTS AND NEBULIZERS

Doctors have long used nasal sprays as a means of getting medication into the body, particularly to the sensitive mucous membranes that line the nasal and sinus passages, both targets for the viruses that cause the common cold and the flu. Influenza live vaccines, FluMist, are already delivered by nasal sprays, as are some antiviral drugs like Zanamivir. Steroid sprays to reduce sinus and lung inflammation are used to treat sinusitis and asthma. Interferon can also be administered as an aerosolized mist to minimize its systemic side effects and produce faster clinical response in the respiratory tract, exactly where the medication is most needed.

Natural medicines including beta-glucan, zinc, and aqueous vitamin A can also be administered by nasal sprays. Compounding pharmacies can make such sprays in normal saline solution for you with a prescription from your doctor.

Reducing lung inflammation is crucial to surviving the flu. Inhaling medications through a nebulizer could make a life or death difference should you or a family member become a victim of pandemic influenza. A nebulizer, sometimes called a "breathing machine," is a medical device that delivers medication in the form of a mist to the airways in the nose and lungs.

You can purchase a nebulizer without a prescription, but since it creates a fine mist, medications must come in liquid form so they can mix easily in water and then be pumped through the device. Your doctor can prescribe medications or have a compounding pharmacy prepare natural substances in liquid form. These include beta-glucan and glutathione. I've previously discussed beta-glucan in detail, so I will talk about glutathione in this section.

Glutathione: Influenza infection induces massive oxidative stress on tissue and cells due to the release of destructive molecules

Beating the Flu

involved in the immune response. Antioxidants like vitamin C, discussed in Chatper 10, are important for fighting the flu and recovering from infection. Glutathione is a naturally occurring powerful antioxidant with anti-influenza activity. However, it's not easily utilized when taken orally. Consuming vitamin C and L-cysteine taken as NAC, both discussed in the previous chapter, can help raise glutathione levels in the body. Since the lung tissue is where it's needed the most, the best way to administer glutathione is in a nebulizer.

The protocol for inhaling glutathione is to use 300-600 mg twice a day in a nebulizer. Each treatment should last five to ten minutes. There are no serious adverse effects associated with inhaling glutathione; however, those with asthma or allergies may experience increased airway restriction and should discontinue if your asthma worsens. Your doctor will have to order glutathione in sterile vials from a compounding pharmacy.

A nebulizer is only as good as the person using it. Learn to use your nebulizer according to the manufacturer's instructions and always follow your physician's written prescribing guidelines and instructions.

INJECTABLE HOMEOPATHIC MEDICINES

Homeopathic combination formulas, some containing herbal extracts as well, have been in use in Europe for decades for the treatment of infections and chronic diseases. They are considered safe, without adverse reactions, and nontoxic. In my clinical experience, they are very effective in managing influenza. Some are available in the United States, while others can be purchased in Germany, Austria, and Switzerland, as well as other European countries. To beat the flu, one ampule is injected intramuscularly three times a week.

Engystol N: Available in an injectable form by prescription and administered by a licensed healthcare practitioner, Engystol N has broad-spectrum antiviral activity and stimulates effective natural immunity.

Gripp-Heel: Like Engystol, this medication is manufactured by

Heel, a German company with manufacturing and distribution in the United States, and comes in tablets or for injection.

Pascotox Forte-Injectopas: This injectable medicine is manufactured by Pascoe Naturmedizin in Germany and is not available in the United States. It contains *Echinacea pallida* root with homeopathics. It is used for symptoms of the flu and secondary infections associated with influenza.

Infekt 1-Injectopas N: Also from Pascoe, this injectable medication contains 12 mg of echinacea in each 2 mL ampoule along with homeopathics such as Aconitum D2, a fever remedy. It can be used to treat upper respiratory infections including the flu. This medication is not available in the United States.

INJECTABLE CHINESE HERBAL MEDICINES

Modern Chinese medicine frequently employs injectable forms of herbal concentrates. Several have use for the treatment of influenza and secondary respiratory tract infections. In China, these medications are given intravenously or injected in minute amounts into acupuncture points. All require prescription and administration by a knowledgeable licensed healthcare practitioner. They may not be available in the United States.

Ban Lan Gen/radix isatidis (*Isatis tinctoria*): This purified extract of isatis is used to stimulate the immune system and to treat viral and minor bacterial infections. It is generally considered safe, but as with all medications, allergic reactions may occur. Due to its ability to inhibit platelets, it should not be given to people taking anticoagulant or antiplatelet drugs such as coumadin and aspirin.

Chai Hu/radix bupleuri (*Bupleurum falcatum*): Influenza viral replication peaks in the body about one to two weeks after infection. Inflammatory reactions, however, continue to occur, especially in the lungs, well after the initial stage of infection has passed and the viral load diminished. It's at this stage that Minor Bupleurum Decoction, the Chinese herbal formula containing bupleurum, and the injectable form are most useful. Bupleurum is a safe herbal medicine but can interact with some drugs, such as steroids and interferon; therefore, it should be used alone.

Beating the Flu

Chuan Xin Lian/herba andrographis *(Andrographis paniculata):* This is the injectable form of andrographis. It has antibacterial and anti-inflammatory activity and is used to treat upper respiratory infections.

BLOOD PURIFICATION: THE HEMOPURIFIER

Theoretically, if viruses and overproduction of immune chemicals could be removed from the blood, the body's own immune power could finish the job of defeating an infection. A blood purification device could be one way to accomplish this when drugs don't work or the patient is overwhelmed with massive viral replication.

One such medical device in development by Aethlon Medical, the Hemopurifier is designed to capture viruses circulating in the blood. It uses dialysis technology and agents that selectively bind viruses, viral proteins, and toxins before they can infect cells or cause tissue damage. The goal is to reduce the viral burden on the body without drugs so the patient's natural immunity can defeat the virus.

Preclinical human blood studies have documented the effectiveness of the Hemopurifier in capturing influenza, hepatitis C, measles, mumps, Ebola, and Marburg viruses, as well as HIV, Orthopoxvirus, and Dengue hemorrhagic fever virus. It also can clear harmful cytokines, the immune chemicals that are responsible for many of the aggressive symptoms related to bird flu infection, from the blood. No adverse events have been reported in the course of use with this device.

12
Outsmart the Flu

The Importance of Personal Preparedness

Infection from influenza virus happens easily and is universal. It occurs by inhaling contaminated air containing viruses spread by coughing and sneezing. A virus can also spread by hand contact and from touching surfaces and objects like cups, phone handsets, keyboards, and doorknobs contaminated by a person suffering from the flu. As a result of nose-blowing and coughing, wet secretions from the nose and lung loaded with flu viruses contaminate the hands of infected people. Unwittingly, they spread the flu in a handshake or inadvertently when they touch an object. Even brief hand contact can transfer the disease. After you touch a contaminated surface or hand, the virus can jump into your body when you scratch your nose or rub your eyes.

Beating the Flu

To catch the flu, you have to be exposed to the virus, so reducing your exposure is the best way not to get sick.

PERSONAL HYGIENE: YOUR BEST CHANCE

Aside from moving to a desert island, personal hygiene and home preparedness may be the two most effective measures in avoiding and treating a super flu. Make it a habit to practice personal hygiene measures. Teach all family members and train your children in proper etiquette when sick. Let's start with the fundamentals.

(!) **Wash your hands:** Keeping viruses away by washing your hands frequently is one of the most important things you can do to avoid catching the flu. Keeping your hands clean also helps prevent passing viruses to someone else. Wash your hands with warm water and a mild detergent soap. Allow plenty of time for the water to rinse the viruses from your skin. A good rule for how long to wash is to sing "Happy Birthday" twice. Ordinary soaps and detergents don't kill influenza virus, but they do help remove dirt and grease that might keep the viruses clinging to the skin, waiting for a chance to make you sick.

If you can't readily wash your hands, use a waterless hand-sanitizing solution. Apply liberally and use a paper towel to dry your hands. Dispose of used towels immediately into a plastic trash bag. Hand wipes can also be used. Remember to use them only once and dispose of them immediately. Don't leave paper towels or hand wipes lying around after use.

(!) **Blow your nose:** Use tissues to blow your nose. Dispose of used tissues properly by placing them in a separate plastic bag before putting them in the trash. Burning tissues may destroy some of the virus, but may release some into the air. Don't burn tissue unless burning trash is approved by the public health department. Do the same with paper towels used to dry your hands, wipe countertops, or clean other surfaces like computer screens and keyboards.

(!) **Clean your clothes:** Wash clothes frequently in hot water with detergent. Dry them at a high temperature. If possible, hang them in the sun, as moving air and sunlight are unfavorable for viruses. Ironing clothes with a steam iron helps to eliminate any lingering germs.

(!) **Dispose of used cloths properly:** Never leave dishcloths, sponges, or rags used to wipe counters lying around. Wash them frequently. After the cloths are dry, microwaving them for 30 seconds destroys most bacteria and viruses. Sanitize sponges and dishcloths by soaking them for ten minutes or longer in a water and bleach solution. Mix 3/4 cup of chlorine bleach in one gallon of water.

(!) **Wipe surfaces:** The flu virus can survive 48 hours or longer on an exposed surface. Keep frequently touched objects like phone handsets, computer keyboards, doorknobs, and other commonly used objects clean. Wipe flat surfaces like countertops, desks, and tables where viruses can land. Use disposable toilet disinfectants, disinfectant spray, or disinfectant wipes, or make your own from bleach. Dispose wipes by placing them in a plastic bag before throwing them in the trash.

(!) **Don't rub your eyes:** Try to keep your hands away from your eyes. Keeping your hands clean helps prevent viruses from getting into your eyes or nose when you do happen to touch them with your hands. Keep long hair tied back, so you don't inadvertently touch your eyes while brushing your hair back.

(!) **Don't linger:** It pulls at our heartstrings to see them sick, but resist sitting at the bedside of a sick family member or other loved one. If you must, stay out of coughing range. The room can be full of viruses hovering in the air and on surfaces. Wear a mask and use gloves to protect yourself. Wearing them is no guarantee that you won't get sick, but it reduces your chances. Don't linger around infected people at work or public events.

Beating the Flu

After shopping, step out of the checkout line if someone is coughing or sneezing near you.

If you've been exposed to the flu and go to work, school, or other public places, you're likely to spread the disease to at least two others. You're contagious when the virus replicates enough to start shedding. That's about a day or two after exposure and lasting five to seven days. During a pandemic in which there are many unknowns about the characteristics of the new virus, the contagious period could be much longer.

(!) **Don't become a germ spreader/Stay home:** A rule of thumb is that when you're coughing and sneezing, you're contagious. As soon as symptoms start, usually a fever, sore throat, and cough, stay home. Don't go to work or to public places like movie theatres. Since the flu spreads rapidly among children and seniors, don't visit schools or nursing homes when you're sick. If you have to go out, or if symptoms start before you can get home, observe the following rules. Turn your head away from others and cover your mouth when you cough. Use a tissue, and avoid using your hand or sleeve to sneeze into. Germs can spread to others in handshakes or by brushing against them. Politely avoid shaking hands. Wash your hands frequently to keep viruses away. If you're at work, have lunch at your desk. Clean up your office before you go home. Wipe your desktop, phone, and computer keyboard with a disinfectant wipe or Lysol spray.

(!) **Don't touch:** It's not bad manners not to shake hands at a meeting. I have a theory that the reason Asians bow instead of shaking hands, or kissing each check as is done in France, is because they knew long ago that viruses spread through touch. Social distance will be acceptable during an influenza pandemic.

(!) **Wear a mask:** To protect others from getting sick, wear a mask if you're coughing. Masks also help protect you from getting sick. No mask is completely reliable, but wearing one helps cut down the spread of infection. Do not clean or reuse masks.

They should be used only once. Discard used masks immediately after use by putting them in a separate plastic bag before disposing of them in the trash. The 3M N95 and N100 are the preferred ones. Surgical masks are a good second choice. Since the influenza virus can pass into your body through the moisture in your eyes, infection control glasses that fit snugly over the mask would be useful if you have to be close to sick people who are coughing and sneezing, such as when tending to a sick family member.

Make sure the mask fits snugly over your face. A poorly fitting mask could allow viruses to sneak by. Tie the strings tightly or position the rubber bands behind your head so the mask is held in place. It should cover your nose, mouth, and chin. Wash your hands before putting on a face mask and after you've disposed of it.

(!) **Wear gloves:** When handling objects touched by a sick person or if you are sick yourself, don't take chances. Wear gloves to protect you and others. Surgical latex or nonlatex disposal gloves are best. Discard them as you would tissue and masks. You can purchase masks and gloves at a medical or surgical supply company or on the Internet.

ACTION TIPS

Chicken and eggs: After the discussion on the benefits of chicken soup, you may wonder if it's safe to eat chicken or eggs during a bird flu epidemic. Though eating well-cooked poultry and eggs isn't considered a risk for infection, handling raw chicken in the preparation process could pose a risk. All utensils, surfaces, and hands that come in contact with raw poultry should be cleaned well with soap and water immediately afterward.

Stay away from poultry farms where chickens, ducks, geese, or turkeys are raised. Don't prepare poultry for consumption unless it's certain that meat or eggs from these birds are safe to eat. Bird flu can infect other birds as well, including parrots and wild birds. It would be wise to stay clear of these birds during an avian flu pandemic.

Watch out for super spreaders: Super spreaders are highly infectious individuals who pass on the disease to scores of others.

127

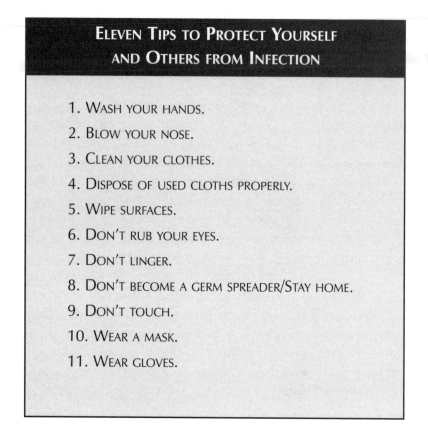

Eleven Tips to Protect Yourself and Others from Infection

1. Wash your hands.

2. Blow your nose.

3. Clean your clothes.

4. Dispose of used cloths properly.

5. Wipe surfaces.

6. Don't rub your eyes.

7. Don't linger.

8. Don't become a germ spreader/Stay home.

9. Don't touch.

10. Wear a mask.

11. Wear gloves.

During the SARS epidemic, one super spreader in a Hong Kong apartment building infected more than 90 people. Because the most infectious 20 percent of individuals are responsible for transmitting most of the disease, avoiding them is critical to remaining disease free. Not only should you cover your nose and mouth when you sneeze, but you should also cover it when in the presence of someone who is coughing or sneezing. Super spreaders are easy to spot. They are constantly coughing and sneezing, and their eyes are usually red and irritated. If you see someone like this, distance yourself.

Avoid flu hot spots: Avoid places where the flu is most likely to spread, such as airports, schools, public transportation systems, and shopping malls. Stay clear of gatherings in closed public buildings with central air and heating systems, through which virus-contaminated air can spread from one part of the building to another. Travel by airplane is particularly important to avoid during a pandemic. If you have to fly or go to public places, you can wear a mask.

Don't travel to pandemic flu hot spots. Unless you're a health-care worker, first responder, or researcher, stay away from known centers of aggressive influenza activity. During a pandemic, these most likely will include all Asian countries.

Nursing homes and hospitals are notorious for passing along infections. If you can, stay out of the hospital and don't frequent nursing homes for the aged. If you have to go to such places, don a mask, wear gloves, and wash your hands before you leave.

Stay informed: Should a pandemic influenza sweep the world, learn as much as you can about the movement and spread of the pandemic. National radio and television will broadcast information. The Internet will provide the most reliable sources of information such as from the World Health Organization (WHO) and Centers for Disease Control (CDC) as well as state government health agencies, universities, and private groups. Besides the global picture, it's necessary to be aware of infection in your community. Listen to local radio and television.

Don't panic: Being prepared by following the measures outlined in this book will reduce your chance of infection. A healthy respect for the power of pandemic influenza is what's needed, not fear. Overreacting due to fear can drive one to do irrational things. Don't panic. Be proactive, not overreactive.

EMERGENCY PREPARATION

Getting ready for an influenza pandemic is a lot like preparing for a hurricane. You have to expect the worst and pray for the best. It's possible that your community may be quarantined or travel restricted in your county. You may have to lock down your home to prevent spread of infection to others if you or a family member is sick, or to protect your family and you from getting infected.

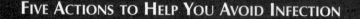

FIVE ACTIONS TO HELP YOU AVOID INFECTION

1. STEER CLEAR OF POULTRY AND PIG FARMS.
2. WATCH OUT FOR SUPER SPREADERS.
3. AVOID INTERNATIONAL FLU HOT SPOTS.
4. STAY INFORMED.
5. DON'T PANIC.

Stockpile food and water: If the Florida hurricanes of 2004 and the hurricanes that hit New Orleans and Mexico in 2005 taught us anything at all about surviving natural disasters, it is that we can't depend on the government, so be well prepared with water and food.

Plant an herb garden: If you're in the southern climates, antiviral and other medicinal herbs will grow all year round. If you're in the north, grow herbs in the summer and dry them for use during the winter. If you can't grow your own, order dried herbs or buy them from your local natural foods store.

Stock up on homeopathic medicines and Chinese herbs: All dried herbs can be kept indefinitely in the freezer. When unopened and kept away from heat and sunlight, homeopathic remedies store well. Store nutritional supplements in the refrigerator.

PREVENTION

True prevention should be proactive rather than reactive. Being knowledgeable and informed and correctly applying what you learned in a timely manner is preferable to beginning treatment when symptoms are out of control. Like the old Chinese saying, it's better to dig the well now rather than wait until you're thirsty.

Lifestyle and supplements: The best prevention is strong viral immunity. You may want to review chapter 8, which discusses how

FIFTEEN PANDEMIC HOME-PREPAREDNESS TIPS

1. Stockpile food (canned and dry goods) and water to last at least three weeks.

2. Store medicines: antibiotics, antivirals, aspirin, acetaminophen.

3. Stockpile natural medicines and dried herbs.

4. Have a supply of gloves and masks.

5. Get a nebulizer and humidifier if you live in a dry climate or have central heating.

6. Keep powdered ginger and mustard on hand to make chest plasters.

7. Store some nose medicines: Vicks, mentholated balms, White Flower Oil, Tiger Balm, and the Swiss product, an Olbas inhaler.

8. Keep flashlights in working order and store extra batteries.

9. Get a clock or watch that runs on batteries.

10. Have a propane grill and enough fuel to last three weeks.

11. Get a battery-operated radio or television.

12. Get a telephone that doesn't require electricity to work.

13. Charge your cell phone.

14. Fill your gas tank.

15. Have markers and poster board at your door for writing messages to emergency workers.

to enhance your immune system. For a detailed exposition on the subject of viruses and the best ways to optimize your immune function, you might find my book *Viral Immunity* valuable.

Strong viral immunity begins with lifestyle choices. Here are the basics: eat a healthful, balanced diet; avoid refined sugar and processed foods; exercise regularly; get enough sleep; take nutritional supplements, especially antioxidants; and use immune-boosting herbal medicines.

Vaccines: Consider getting a flu shot for ordinary flu. During a pandemic, ordinary influenza will also circulate and you could catch both at the same time. If a safe vaccine is produced for pandemic influenza, you may want to get that as well, if it's available. For people with existing lung diseases and the elderly, consider getting the pneumonia vaccination.

VACCINATION OPTIONS

- ✦ Seasonal flu shot
- ✦ Pandemic flu shot
- ✦ Pneumonia shot

RECOGNITION OF FLU SYMPTOMS

Knowing the characteristics of the flu is essential for recognition of symptoms. Review chapters 3 and 4 to learn about influenza and how viruses alter their genes, like a chameleon changes color to survive. I discussed the difference between a cold and the flu and between ordinary flu and pandemic flu earlier in the book. It may be a good time to reread those sections now.

If you or a family member becomes sick, evaluate symptoms early. Is it a cold or the flu? If others in your school, at work, or in your community have become sick with the bird flu, you most likely have been exposed and the chances that you've been infected are high. If you have a fever, sore throat, and cough, it's very likely that you have the flu. Isolate yourself from others in the house. Everyone should wear a mask and gloves when in your room. Keep all surfaces wiped clean. Weather permitting, keep a window open to allow fresh air into the room and keep the room warm. Influenza viruses like cool dark places, and your lungs don't work as well in dry stuffy air. Let some sunshine in, if you can and it's not too cold outside to do so.

EARLY INTERVENTION

If you suspect you've become infected, start treatment early. Take vitamin C, or if you're already taking this important antioxidant and virus-fighting nutrient, increase the dosage to 1,500 mg every few hours. If this amount causes intestinal gas, bloating, or diarrhea, back off to 500 mg per dose. Keep up your nutrition with healthy foods and take a multiple vitamin and mineral supplement. Take at least 30 mg of zinc daily. Drink enough water to stay hydrated. Humidify your room or inhale steam to keep your airways moist. Rest and get in some extra sleep to tune up your immune system.

Inhaling steam moistens nasal passages and upper airways to the lungs and helps relieve congestion. Influenza viruses and those that cause the common cold don't like warm steam, but there is little scientific evidence that it reduces viral shedding in the nasal passages. It's a home remedy with merit, however, and a history as old as the use of hot rocks to boil water. To create steam, boil water on the stove, and when it is robustly steaming, remove the pot or kettle from the stove and put it on the floor or a low table. Sit with your head over the pot, with a towel over your head to trap the steam, and inhale deeply. The water should be hot, but not boiling, so the steam doesn't burn your face.

A simple method that is safe and works well with infants and small children is to steam up the bathroom by letting the shower run with hot water only. Lay a towel along the bottom of the door to keep the steam in and cold air out. Inhaling the moisture in a steamy bathroom is refreshing as well as helpful for relieving congestion. Do not sit directly under the shower or you may get burned.

Beating the Flu

To clear the nose and lungs so you can breathe better, add a half-teaspoon of Vicks or other menthol rub, one to two drops of eucalyptus oil, or a few slices of fresh ginger to the boiling water or sprinkle in the shower to enhance the decongestant effect. Mentholated inhalers help open clogged sinuses. Try Vicks, White Flower Oil, Tiger Balm, or Olbas.

Another way to clear the nasal passages is with a saltwater rinse. Mix 1/4 teaspoon salt in 8 ounces of warm water. If saltwater alone is too irritating to sensitive nasal membranes, add 1/4 teaspoon baking soda. Sterile water is best. If you don't have some, boil the water to sterilize it. Wait until it cools before mixing in the salt. You know you have the right amount of salt if it tastes like tears. Use a bulb syringe to squirt body-temperature water into your nose. You can also use a ceramic neti pot. Hold one nostril closed by applying light finger pressure while squirting the salt mixture into the other nostril. Let it drain. Repeat two to three times, then treat the other nostril.

For the sore throat that often comes early and makes it hard to swallow when you have the flu, start gargling with warm saltwater or lemon and honey water. Drinking a cup of warm water with a few drops of myrrh or propolis tincture or liquid grapefruit seed extract added to it can work wonders on inflamed tonsils and sensitive throat membranes. For severe sore throat, you may have to gargle every 30 minutes to get relief.

Your grandmother's old-fashioned remedies might come to the rescue. Try a ginger or mustard chest plaster to lessen coughing, open chest congestion, and ease breathing. Don't use them on young children or people with sensitive skin as they can sting and cause an uncomfortable burning sensation. To make a plaster, combine 4 teaspoons of flour with 2 teaspoons of olive oil and 1 tablespoon of dry mustard or ginger powder, and mix in lukewarm water to form a paste. Spread the paste on a thin clean cloth and place on chest for 20 minutes. After you take the plaster off, rub the chest with camphorated oil or Vicks and cover with a warm fabric such as flannel or a towel.

When to call your doctor: It's likely that during a super flu pandemic, phone hotlines will be set up to help direct you to the right

SORE THROAT SOLUTIONS

✧ **ONION AND HONEY:** Slice one whole white or yellow onion and spread the slices on a thin baking dish; cover with honey. Warm in the oven at 150°F for 1 hour. Remove the onions and mix 1 tablespoon of the honey in 1 cup of hot water.

✧ **MYRRH AND/OR PROPOLIS:** Mix 1/3 to 1 teaspoon of myrrh or propolis tincture, or combine them, in 1/2 cup of warm water. Gargle twice daily.

✧ **RASPBERRY LEAVES AND LEMON:** Steep 1 tablespoon of dry raspberry leaves with a little fresh lemon juice in 2 cups of hot water; mix with 1 teaspoon of honey. Let the mixture cool to room temperature before gargling.

✧ **WARM SALTWATER:** Mix 1/3 teaspoon of table or sea salt into 1 cup of warm water. It should not be too salty but taste about the salinity of tears. Use as a mouth rinse and gargle as needed to control symptoms.

✧ **ZINC LOZENGES:** Suck on zinc lozenges as needed to control symptoms. Don't exceed 30 mg per day.

treatment and to decide whether you should go to the hospital. Your local community hospital and larger medical groups may have their own triage system, a method of prioritizing medical emergencies. Call if you have a high fever, have difficulty breathing, relentless coughing, or thick dark-colored or blood-tinged mucus.

TIPS FOR EARLY TREATMENT

- ❖ Vitamin C: 1,500 mg every 2–3 hours.
- ❖ Zinc: 30 mg daily or zinc lozenges.
- ❖ Drink 8–10 glasses of water daily.
- ❖ Humidify your room or inhale steam.
- ❖ Rinse your mouth and gargle with warm saltwater.
- ❖ Inhale Olbas to relieve a stuffy nose.
- ❖ Get extra rest and enough sleep.

When to go to the hospital: Should a super flu cripple the economy, your local hospital will likely be overwhelmed with cases. Field hospitals might be in place to handle less serious cases. Schools and other public buildings might be converted into temporary clinics. Ventilators and oxygen to assist breathing will be in short supply. Go to the hospital if your doctor directs you to do so. There are times, however, when you should go directly to the emergency room. These include when an infant has a very high fever and when any individual has extreme difficulty breathing, severe headache, and unrelenting vomiting and diarrhea.

KNOW THE RIGHT TREATMENT

To beat the flu, you have to use the right treatment at the right time. Starting early with natural medicines is by far better than waiting until you're so sick you can't get out of bed.

When to start an antiviral drug: If you've stockpiled Tamiflu or another antiviral drug, to be effective it must be taken within the first 48 hours after appearance of symptoms. It is not likely to make a difference if you've had symptoms for longer than a few days. An antiviral drug can also be used preventively if you've been exposed. The bottom line for antiviral drugs is the sooner the better.

The average dosage of Tamiflu for children older than 13 and adults is 75 mg twice daily for five days, taken with food to prevent stomach upset. Severe and hospitalized cases require 150 mg twice daily for ten to 14 days. If you've been exposed, the recommended dosage is 75 mg daily for seven days. These are average recommended dosages, but medical opinion changes; therefore consult with your prescribing physician for the most current information. You can also find information on the CDC and WHO websites.

When to take antibiotics: If you've stockpiled antibiotics, only use them if a proven bacterial infection is present. Upper respiratory tract infections caused by viruses won't respond to antibiotics. Even green-colored phlegm, once thought to be a sign of bacterial breeding in the mucus, may not be helped by taking antibiotics. Inappropriate use of antibiotics can disrupt your natural immune balance enough to allow for increased incidence of respiratory tract infections.

Young children, immune-compromised patients, the elderly, and those with underlying respiratory tract disease are most likely to develop bacterial infections secondary to influenza. These people may need antibiotics to prevent life-threatening infection. Delaying taking antibiotics for a few days, however, until you're sure they're necessary, won't make a significant difference to their effectiveness.

The best way to diagnose a bacterial infection is through a throat or sputum culture. A high white-blood-cell count, as determined by a blook test, is a signal that there's an infection in the body. Getting a culture or laboratory test may take too long, however, and laboratories may be swamped with testing. You may have to rely on your own or your doctor's good judgment.

Here are some signs and symptoms to consider when determining if you have a bacterial infection severe enough to warrant taking an antibiotic. A temperature of 100–102°F is normal in the first few days of influenza. If fever lasts longer than a few days, is above 102°F, or returns after having subsided, a bacterial infection may be present. If your symptoms don't improve after two weeks or worsen considerably during the first seven to ten days, and high fever and severe cough are present, you may need an antibiotic. For public safety during an influenza pandemic, however, antibiotic use should be curbed. The bottom line for antibiotics is that they are best pre- scribed by a knowledgeable physician.

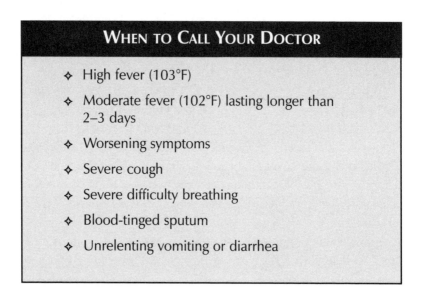

WHEN TO CALL YOUR DOCTOR

✦ High fever (103°F)

✦ Moderate fever (102°F) lasting longer than 2–3 days

✦ Worsening symptoms

✦ Severe cough

✦ Severe difficulty breathing

✦ Blood-tinged sputum

✦ Unrelenting vomiting or diarrhea

Steroids: Corticosteroid drugs like prednisone profoundly lower inflammation in the lungs. However, because of their severe adverse potential, steroid prescribing should be left to a medical profes- sional. Consider natural anti-inflammatory alternatives:

CAT'S CLAW: 1,000 MG THREE TIMES DAILY.

GINGER: MAKE A TEA FROM 4–5 SLICES OF FRESH GINGER PER CUP OF HOT WATER. DRINK 1 CUP THREE TIMES DAILY.

QUERCETIN: 500 MG THREE TIMES DAILY.

Dehydration: As a consequence of high fever, especially when accompanied by sweating, vomiting, and diarrhea, you can lose a large volume of body fluid. If fluid is not replaced, you become dehydrated. In its most severe form, dehydration can result in death from kidney failure. Symptoms include extreme weakness, fainting, and headache. Since these also are also symptoms of the flu, however, watch for these specific signs: very dry mouth and tongue, loss of skin elasticity, and decreased urination and urine that is dark brown in color. During severe dehydration, death can come in a matter of days. Don't wait until you (or a family member) become dehydrated; start giving fluids early on when you have the flu.

Drinking water is the best way to replace fluids. Herbal teas, soups, green coconut water, fruit and vegetable juices, and thin gruel made from oats and rice or other grains are flavorful ways of replacing fluids, and they have the added benefit of replacing lost minerals. Plain water and even juices, teas, broths, or milk don't replenish electrolytes sufficiently when you're very sick.

When someone becomes dehydrated, they not only lose water, but electrolytes as well. These are salts of sodium, chloride, potassium, and other minerals that help maintain fluid balance in the body. In the hospital, fluids and electrolytes are replaced intravenously. During pandemic influenza, however, you may not be able to get to the hospital or they may be too crowded to treat you. Prepare for such an event by having fluid and electrolyte replacement beverages at home.

Commercial effervescent vitamin C powder with minerals mixed in water is a good way to get your antioxidants, electrolytes, and the bicarbonate that helps reduce acidity in the body. Sports drinks like Gatorade are helpful because they not only help replace fluids and electrolytes, but also contain sugar to keep glucose levels normal. If you don't eat for several days, your body's glucose (blood sugar) levels drop and you become weaker. This is important because when sick with the flu, you have no appetite or can't keep food down if you're vomiting.

You can purchase packets of oral rehydration solution (ORS) that readily reconstitutes in water or you can make your own from water, ordinary table salt (sodium chloride), and sugar or honey. Molasses and raw sugar contain potassium and may be better than white sugar. Orange juice also contains potassium. For severe dehydration, take fluids a teaspoon at a time, if necessary, until you've consumed two to three quarts per day. A good measure of how successful you are in replacing fluids is when you start to urinate again. When you are urinating four to five times daily and the color is clear, you are out of danger from dehydration.

HOMEMADE ORAL REHYDRATION SOLUTION

1/2 teaspoon salt

1/2 teaspoon baking soda

3 tablespoons sugar

Combine the ingredients and stir into one quart of pure bottled or boiled water.

If fever continues for several days, or there is severe unrelenting vomiting or diarrhea, call your doctor or go to the nearest emergency room. You may need intravenous fluids and electrolytes.

Oxygen and ventilators: For severe respiratory distress, mechanical breathing machines and oxygen are lifesaving. During a pandemic, however, there will not be enough to go around. Therefore, only the most critically ill will receive ventilators. If you or a family member has chronic respiratory disease, request your doctor to write a prescription for a portable home oxygen tank. Learn to use it properly. During a pandemic, if you or someone in your family is having extreme difficulty breathing, call your doctor or go to the nearest emergency room.

Supportive care: Over-the-counter medicines offer relief for some of the symptoms of influenza but don't cure it. They are not recommended as medicines to beat the flu, but to lessen some of the symptoms.

Nonsteroidal anti-inflammatory medications such as ibuprofen (Advil) can help reduce inflammation and are useful in treating headache and muscle soreness. Aspirin also has anti-inflammatory along with pain-relieving properties and can be used for adults. Don't give aspirin to children who have the flu.

Acetaminophen (Tylenol) can be taken to control fever, lessen the aches and pains associated with the flu, and soften headache pressure. Though a common ingredient in many cold and flu remedies, acetaminophen can cause liver damage.

To protect your liver, take N-acetyl-L-cysteine (NAC), which is made in the body for the purpose of enhancing the production of the molecule glutathione, a powerful antioxidant. NAC has anti-inflammatory and antiviral properties, and helps break up thick mucus so you can breathe better. Take 500 mg three times daily when you have the flu.

Pseudoephedrine (Sudafed) is helpful for relieving nasal congestion. Expectorants and cough suppressants (Robitussin DM) and

OVER-THE-COUNTER AIDS FOR WHEN YOU HAVE THE FLU

- ✧ Ibuprofen: for pain and inflammation
- ✧ Aspirin: for fever, pain, and inflammation (do not give to children)
- ✧ Acetaminophen: for fever and pain
- ✧ Pseudoephedrine: to relieve nasal congestion
- ✧ Expectorants and cough suppressants: to get rid of mucus and control coughing
- ✧ Guaifenesin: to thin mucus

drugs that thin phlegm (e.g., guaifenesin) can help you get sleep by reducing your coughing and excess mucus in your airways.

Follow your doctor's advice when taking these medications and read the directions on the package for dosages. Take them as recommended. Don't take them for longer than seven days without a healthcare practitioner's supervision or advice from your pharmacist.

13
Family Matters

Taking Care of Children and Seniors

Since pandemic influenza tends to be highly contagious, it's not uncommon for a family, town, or everyone in a community to get sick. Depending on individual viral immunity, family members will start to come down with the flu as early as two to three days after the first person started having symptoms. It only takes one infected member to bring the flu home.

As you recall, there are no symptoms the first few days after being exposed. In a pandemic strain, this symptom-free period, when the virus is incubating in your tissues, can last as long as a week. Meanwhile, the virus is taking hold in your body and you are becoming contagious.

Once you start coughing, you are very contagious. Your family can become sick unless you take preventive measures. Even if every member eventually catches the flu, it's better if you don't all get sick at the same time.

Severe flu can make you so sick that if you're the family caretaker, you can't get out of bed to attend to your children. Each member should have a designated duty should you fall ill.

Follow the measures in the previous chapter on personal preparedness. Teach everyone in your family proper hygiene and how to avoid catching the flu when in public places. In addition to the strategies I outline in chapters 8 through 11, in this chapter I discuss matters of special significance for children and the elderly. Here's a review of some of the key points.

Isolation: Though not easy to accomplish in a large family, isolation may be necessary to slow down the spread of infection. Wear a mask when in the room, not just by the sickbed. Viral particles will be thick in the air and on surfaces. Wear gloves when wiping down surfaces and cleaning. Wash your hands thoroughly with soap and warm water. Only sick family members should sleep in the same bed. Kissing is out until you're completely well.

Ventilation: Keep air moving by cracking a window or running a portable fan on the lowest setting. Good ventilation assists breathing and is unfavorable to survival of influenza virus. If weather permits, keep a window open and let the sunshine in during the daytime hours. Keep the room warm at night. Use a humidifier if the air is too dry.

Personal protection: Follow the same principles for personal protection discussed in the previous chapter and teach them to your family. Wash hands correctly. Don't share towels, toothbrushes, or personal items. Keep long hair tied back so you don't inadvertently touch your eyes while brushing back your loose hair. Cover your mouth and nose when you cough or sneeze. Discard tissue properly. Keep surfaces like kitchen counters and desktops and frequently used surfaces like phone handsets and computer keyboards wiped down with a disinfectant solution. Discard paper towels properly.

Keep your family members strong: Make sure they get enough rest and sound sleep. When sleeping, don't wake them to give them medications. The immune benefits of deep sleep far outweigh the need for drugs or vitamins. They can take their medicine when awake. Provide a healthful diet with plenty of fresh fruits and vegetables, fresh squeezed orange juice, herbal teas, and soups. Follow a nutritional supplement plan and the advice for immune building in the previous two chapters.

PROTECTING YOUR CHILDREN

The H5N1 bird flu has been particularly hard on children. Those younger than 15 have been most commonly infected and have the highest death rate. For nuisance viruses such as ordinary influenza or chickenpox, getting repeated exposure while young strengthens immunity against future infection. Whereas repeated exposure is good practice for ordinary flu and common childhood viruses, it's bad news for pandemic influenza.

Since infection during a pandemic can be fatal in small children, protect them from getting sick. No one is immune from a new influenza strain; therefore the best prevention is complete protection. That's difficult, however, because children are the perfect carriers and spreaders of flu. They mingle closely, don't wipe their runny noses, cough without covering their mouths, and touch everything in sight. If at all possible, keep children from mingling with each other.

Here are some additional tips for protecting your children from the flu and what to do should they get sick.

At school or day care: Keep all surfaces and door handles wiped down. Machine-wash toys such as stuffed animals in hot water and detergent. Wipe plastic and wooden toys with bleach solution or sanitized wipes. Let them air dry and, if possible, leave them in the sun to dry. Make sure all children wash their hands frequently and correctly.

At home: Small children run through the house touching everything in their path. If you have little ones at home, keep surfaces at child level wiped clean. Make sure all children wash their hands thoroughly with soap and warm water. You should wash your hands more frequently when caring for children. Teach them to use tissues to cover their mouths and noses when coughing or sneezing. Dispose of used tissue carefully.

Keep them hydrated: The lives of many infants and children will be saved during a super flu pandemic by preventing dehydration. You can stockpile premixed commercial pediatric hydration solutions purchased from your local drugstore or stockpile enough of the ingredients needed to make your own.

Once a fever starts, make sure your child gets fluid in the form of water, sweetened herbal teas, juices, and even sodas without caffeine like ginger ale or 7-Up. Vegetable soups and gruel made from grains are helpful because they contain nutrients. Warm water with lemon and honey is also helpful. If your child is vomiting or has diarrhea, keep the fluids going for three to four days. For severe dehydration, soups, sodas, milk, and plain water are not enough. Follow the recipe to make your own ORS beverage. Adjust the taste as needed so your child will drink it. If necessary, let the child drink from a straw or, using a teaspoon, gently help him or her to drink one spoonful at a time. Take your child to the hospital if he or she has a high fever for more than two days or becomes severely dehydrated.

Immune boosting for kids: Small children and young teens need immune enhancing as much as or more than adults do. The best ones for them are colostrum and beta-glucan. These are safe and nontoxic, and can be mixed into juice, apple sauce, or yogurt if the child can't swallow capsules. You can also make a fruit smoothie by blending fruits and berries of your choice with ice, rice or soy milk, one tablespoon of whey protein powder, colostrum, and beta-glucan. Sweeten with honey or brown sugar. Recommended dosages for immune boosting for kids are:

COLOSTRUM: 450 MG TWICE DAILY.

BETA-GLUCAN: 100 MG TWICE DAILY.

Vitamins for kids: Children of all ages can benefit from a multiple vitamin and mineral supplement. Extra vitamin C is also valuable. Recommended dosages are:

CHILDREN'S MULTIPLE VITAMIN AND MINERAL: TAKE WITH
  MEALS.
VITAMIN C: 100 TO 250 MG AS A CHEWABLE TABLET 3–4
  TIMES DAILY.
ZINC LOZENGES: SUCK ON ONE LOZENGE SEVERAL TIMES
  DAILY.

Herbs for kids: Herbal medicines can be safely used for children. The dosage is generally half of the recommended adult amount for children between ages 6 and 14. Small children can take one-quarter of the adult dose. Teenagers older than 14 can take the recommended average adult dosage. Swallowing capsules or tablets can be difficult for kids, so try tinctures mixed in juice:

ECHINACEA TINCTURE: TAKE 1/3 TEASPOON EVERY 3
  HOURS.
ELDERBERRY TINCTURE: TAKE 1/3 TEASPOON EVERY 3
  HOURS.
GE XIAN WENG: DISSOLVE ONE PACKAGE IN A CUP OF
  HOT WATER.

These herbs are considered safe and nontoxic for children, nursing mothers, and pregnant women. The Chinese herbal tea *ge xian weng* is an instant granule that readily dissolves in water and is presweetened. None of these herbs should be taken for longer than four weeks.

Homeopathics for kids: Medicines that are pleasant tasting and dissolve in the mouth are easy to take. Since the potency of homeopathic medicines is very low, they are completely safe for infants and young children. They are best taken every 30 minutes during an acute infection and when there is fever. Otherwise, dosage is the same as for adults and medicines are taken every three to four hours until symptoms abate. Recommended homeopathic medicines for children are:

GRIPP-HEEL TABLETS: DISSOLVE 1 TABLET IN THE MOUTH
  EVERY 15 MINUTES FOR ACUTE SYMPTOMS.

Beating the Flu

ENGYSTOL N TABLETS: DISSOLVE 1 TABLET IN THE MOUTH
EVERY 15 MINUTES FOR ACUTE SYMPTOMS.

CARE AND TREATMENT OF SENIORS

In civilized society, the strong and healthy are supposed to protect the weak, infirm, and elderly. Our version of protecting seniors,
however, is to warehouse them in facilities that keep them alive but
don't enhance their health or promote well-being. Nursing homes
are perfect breeding grounds for illness, including pneumonia and
diarrheal disease. During flu season, infection can spread through a
nursing home with impunity. The very old are mainly bedridden
and have poor heart and lung function. Even mild seasonal
influenza is life-threatening for them. Many facilities are dark inside
and air doesn't circulate well. Maintaining good ventilation and
allowing the sun in helps reduce infection.

During a flu pandemic, wear gloves and a mask when visiting a
nursing home. Wash your hands before leaving and again on return-

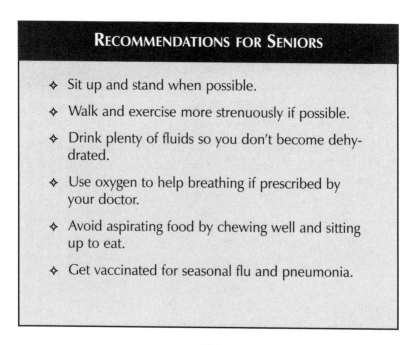

RECOMMENDATIONS FOR SENIORS

✦ Sit up and stand when possible.

✦ Walk and exercise more strenuously if possible.

✦ Drink plenty of fluids so you don't become dehydrated.

✦ Use oxygen to help breathing if prescribed by
  your doctor.

✦ Avoid aspirating food by chewing well and sitting
  up to eat.

✦ Get vaccinated for seasonal flu and pneumonia.

ing home or to work. Don't linger if you don't have to and don't touch surfaces like door handles and phone handsets. Don't visit if you're sick.

Natural medicines for seniors: Vitamins, minerals, immune-boosting substances, herbs, and DHEA can be very helpful to the elderly in promoting health and beating the flu. As soon as fall arrives, start preparing for the winter flu season. Take a multiple vitamin and mineral without iron with each meal. Consider taking ginseng or astragalus to promote health, stamina, and viral immunity. Take colostrum, beta-glucan, and other immune-boosting supplements. Take extra vitamin C and zinc. Follow the recommendations in this book on how to take natural medicines for beating the flu. For frail, older people, reduce the dosage by half.

14
Survive and Recover

A Plan to Beat the Flu

The whole point of this book is to help you treat influenza successfully, manage complications effectively, and survive a super flu pandemic. It is meant to inform you about the benefits and risks of vaccination and drugs so, should you need to use them, your chances of experiencing adverse effects are lessened. It teaches you how to use a physician's services judiciously and suggests some alternative natural medicines that your doctor may not know about but that could save your life.

Since no one is immune to pandemic influenza, if you are exposed, you will get infected. But if you are to get sick, managing infection properly can reduce the severity of the illness, shorten the duration, and minimize complications. The evidence from the growing scientific research base, mounting clinical reports, and the

Beating the Flu

SARS experience strongly points to the fact that using natural medicines offers protection and helps reduce the intensity of infection. Indiscriminate popping of health pills simultaneously with prescription and over-the-counter drugs is a poor mix, however. Choose your medications wisely and take them as directed.

In my practice, I've used all of the natural medicines discussed in this book to treat acute infections and chronic viral illness. In more than 20 years of clinical practice, I've had not one adverse event. Occasionally, patients get nauseous from taking too many pills at once, experience abdominal bloating, or have a bout of diarrhea. But even that's uncommon. I'm cautious about mixing herbal medicine with drugs, but as a rule of thumb, nutritional supplements are safe when taken in the recommended dosages.

Taking the lead from nature when using natural medicines to beat the flu, I've leaned from decades of clinical practice that it's best to approach a disease from multiple angles simultaneously. If done expertly, this approach creates a therapeutic synergism where the sum of the treatment is greater than the individual components. When out to beat the flu, there are specific treatment categories that are essential, including immune enhancement, management of inflammation, supportive nutrition and supplementation with vitamins and minerals, protection of the lungs, as well as the use of natural antiviral medicines.

I would like to believe that vaccines and antiviral drugs will work, but it's hard for me to trust that big pharmaceutical companies, the same ones that brought us Vioxx and didn't warn us about the cancer-causing potential of synthetic estrogen when it was known for decades, have our best interests in mind. American doctors are not well prepared to treat infectious disease, they depend on drug sales reps to inform them about new drugs, and they will be overwhelmed with cases should a pandemic occur. If the government and corporate first choice—immunization and antiviral drugs—is suspect, doesn't it make sense to have a backup—Plan B?

A COMPREHENSIVE APPROACH

In reviewing the research and clinical evidence on all of the natural medicines, homeopathic remedies, and nutritional supplements that might be useful in treating the flu, I've chosen the best and offer here a plan to help you beat the flu. In this section, I identify six main aspects to address when treating pandemic influenza using natural medicines. In the following section of this chapter, I present five natural antiviral prescriptions. If the plan is followed correctly and in a timely manner, I believe it will increase your chances for survival and recovery.

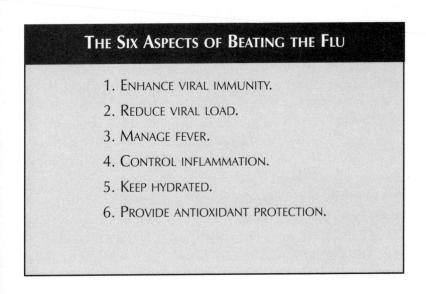

THE SIX ASPECTS OF BEATING THE FLU

1. ENHANCE VIRAL IMMUNITY.

2. REDUCE VIRAL LOAD.

3. MANAGE FEVER.

4. CONTROL INFLAMMATION.

5. KEEP HYDRATED.

6. PROVIDE ANTIOXIDANT PROTECTION.

1. Enhance viral immunity. Begin building your viral immunity in the fall. Don't wait for the flu to hit. This way, when flu season begins in winter and peaks in the spring, you're ready.

Strong viral immunity is particularly important for the elderly, for children, if you have existing lung disease, or if you are easily susceptible to colds and ordinary flu. Study the information in chapter 8 and, for more details, read my book *Viral Immunity*.

Beating the Flu

It's imperative that you not overstimulate your immune system in the mistaken belief that you can defeat a pandemic influenza strain. Though important for preventing the frequency of the common cold and ordinary flu, aggressive defenses are responsible for much of the tissue damage associated with the bird flu infection, as it was with SARS. The regimen I recommend attacks influenza on several fronts and is careful not to overstimulate the immune system.

Whatever time of year it is, begin taking nutritional supplements if you've been exposed to the flu or work in a high-risk environment like a hospital, airport, or public building. If a pandemic is to break out, prophylactic treatment with natural medicines is a safe and effective way to prevent serious infection.

2. Reduce viral load. There are three ways to lower the viral load. The first is with antiviral drugs. They don't always help, however, and are not that effective even when they do. Drugs can also cause significant adverse events. In addition, they exert immune pressure on the virus, causing it to mutate. Eventually, antiviral drugs won't be effective at all as the virus learns ways to resist their pharmacological action.

The second way is with blood purification devices and therapies. I introduced one such device, the Hemopurifier, in chapter 11. Ozone therapy and intravenous hydrogen peroxide are other ways of reducing the viral load in your blood. These services require a specially trained, skilled physician to administer. Before the pandemic comes, inquire if your local hospital is equipped with blood purification devices or has a plan to purchase them. Find out which physicians in your community employ ozone or intravenous hydrogen peroxide therapy in their practice of medicine.

Natural antiviral medicines, the third way to reduce viral load, can slow down replication and reduce the number of viruses in the body, making it easier for your immune system to do its job more effectively. Now would be a good time to reread chapter 10, in which I discuss herbal antiviral medicines.

3. Manage fever. Fever is a natural response to infection and is associated with inflammation. The average body temperature for a healthy person is 98.6°F (37°C). Once the temperature rises close to or higher than 100°F, feverish sensations usually appear. The symptoms of fever include flushing, chills, sweating, and aching joints and muscles.

As body temperature rises with high fever (102–104°F), symptoms intensify, with severe chills, profuse sweating, mental disorientation, and even hallucinations. Unless managed, high fever can cause permanent tissue damage or lead to life-threatening dehydration. Reread chapter 12 to learn when to call your doctor or go to the hospital.

You can manage mild fevers at home with herbal teas and homeopathic medicines. Elderberry (*Sambucus nigra*) or yarrow (*Achilles millefolium*) drunk as an infusion is a good herbal choice. Aconite and Belladona (6–12X potency) are useful homeopathic remedies for controlling fever. The prepared Chinese herbal remedies *yin chiao chieh tu pien* or *ban lan gen chong ji* have long been used to treat fever and viral infection. Review the resources in the back of the book for companies that sell these products.

Cool compresses or tepid baths help keep the heat down. Contrary to popular opinion, rubbing alcohol should not be used to control fever. It can absorb through the skin and cause toxic effects in the body. Don't pile on the blankets if you have chills. Bundling up can cause body temperature to rise. Acetaminophen helps lower fever. Aspirin is useful, but only for adults. Don't give children aspirin when they have the flu. Follow your doctor's dosing directions or those on the product label. You may want to study the section on fever in my book *Viral Immunity*.

4. Control inflammation. SARS and H5N1 bird flu infection has been characterized by massive inflammation in the lungs and other tissues. Steroid drugs are effective in dousing the flames; however, they pose serious health threats when used in the high dosages necessary to quell inflammation caused by influenza. Therefore it's imperative that you understand the importance of managing inflammation with natural medicines. I've devoted an entire chapter in *Viral Immunity* to this crucial factor in beating the flu.

Here are some of the highlights for effectively managing inflammation. Rest and get more sleep. Eat a healthful, balanced diet rich in fresh organic vegetables and omega-3 fatty acids from fish oils. Reduce acidity and increase alkalinity. Use buffered vitamin C rather than pure ascorbic acid. In the first phase of an acute infection, drink wheat grass juice or fresh mixed-green vegetable juices, or take spirulina, barley green, or chlorella powder mixed in water. A fast way to reduce acidity during active infection is to take one-quarter teaspoon of sodium and potassium bicarbonate every two hours. Nutrients that help control inflammation include quercetin, selenium, and lipoic acid.

5. Keep hydrated. Drink water and herbal teas, and keep your electrolytes strong right from the start. Don't allow yourself to get dehydrated. Remember, if you have a fever and are sweating, you're going to lose fluids faster than normal. Read more about dehydration and replacing fluids in chapter 12.

6. Provide antioxidant protection. Viral infection causes massive cellular and major tissue damage, especially in the lungs. As cells and tissues are destroyed, they undergo advanced oxidative changes. During acute infection, the body's repair mechanisms can't keep up with the rate of damage. Providing the body with extra antioxidants in food and supplements helps minimize cell damage and promotes tissue repair. Fruits and vegetables contain natural antioxidants, as do herbal teas and green juices. Examples of antioxidant nutrients include vitamins C and E and the minerals zinc and selenium.

ANTI-FLU PRESCRIPTION 1:
A HEALTHY FOUNDATION

- **BETA-GLUCAN:** 500 MG THREE TIMES DAILY
- **CORDYCEPS:** 250 MG THREE TIMES DAILY
- **NAC:** 250 MG THREE TIMES DAILY
- **QUERCETIN:** 250 MG THREE TIMES DAILY
- **SELENIUM:** 400 MCG DAILY
- **SPIRULINA:** 1,500 MG DAILY
- **VITAMIN A:** 20,000 IU DAILY
- **VITAMIN C:** 1,000 THREE TIMES DAILY
- **ZINC:** 30 MG DAILY

Start taking these supplements in the fall or at the first evidence that a pandemic has started. Once you've initiated my plan by taking the immune-building and antioxidant medications in Anti-Flu Prescription 1, you've put the foundation in place for beating the flu. However, that's just the beginning.

At the first signs of symptoms, begin taking the natural antiviral medicines listed in Prescription 2. Don't wait. Even if you can't distinguish between a cold or flu, or ordinary flu and pandemic flu, starting early with natural medicines is safe. Also, unlike pharmaceutical antiviral drugs, natural medicines are less likely to cause viral mutation, so you won't be contributing to a worse pandemic scenario.

Choose one or more of the herbal and homeopathic medications listed above. To treat a viral infection and boost immunity, choose echinacea. If you have a secondary bacterial infection, use garlic. For the early stages of infection with fever, select elderberry. For children, use elderberry tea and Oscillococcinum.

Since these are safe medications without adverse effects, start

ANTI-FLU PRESCRIPTION 2: EARLY TREATMENT	
• **GARLIC:**	250 MG TWICE DAILY
• **ELDERBERRY:**	700 MG TWICE DAILY
• **ECHINACEA TINCTURE:**	1 TEASPOON THREE TIMES DAILY IN WATER
• **OSCILLOCOCCINUM:**	AS DIRECTED ON INSTRUCTIONS

early and continue for several weeks or even months. If your symptoms clear in a week to ten days, most likely you only had a cold or ordinary flu, and can discontinue taking them.

If you've been infected by pandemic influenza, you have to treat it aggressively and immediately. This is not the time to shop for medicine, so it is to be hoped that you've already stockpiled some along with protective gear such as masks. Reread and study chapter 12 now, before you become sick, to learn what supplies you need to have on hand.

If you're taking pharmaceutical drugs, it's generally safe to take nutritional supplements and homeopathic medicines at the same time. Though there is the possibility of herb-drug interactions, little is known about how oseltamivir may respond when herbs are taken at the same time. Reread the information for each herb in this book, and for updated information, consult your doctor, pharmacist, or pharmacologist at your local hospital or one affiliated with a medical school.

To treat acute illness effectively, ratchet up your program from infection protection to maximum intervention. The first step is to increase the dosages of the natural medications listed in Anti-Flu Prescriptions 1 and 2. For the average adult, the rule of thumb is to double or even triple the recommended dosages. For children's doses, which are smaller, see the previous chapter.

Chinese medicines can play a significant role in this phase of treatment. Take the Chinese herbs as recommended in chapter 10

ANTI-FLU PRESCRIPTION 3:
MAXIMUM INTERVENTION

- **BETA-GLUCAN:** 1,500 MG FOUR TIMES DAILY
- **CORDYCEPS:** 1,500 MG FOUR TIMES DAILY
- **SPIRULINA:** 2,500 MG TWICE DAILY
- **VITAMIN C:** 1,500 MG FOUR TIMES DAILY
- **ZINC:** 30 MG TWICE DAILY
- **SELENIUM:** 400 MCG TWICE DAILY
- **QUERCETIN:** 500 MG FOUR TIMES DAILY
- **NAC:** 1,000 MG FOUR TIMES DAILY
- **VITAMIN A:** 20,000 IU TWICE DAILY
- **GARLIC:** 500 MG FOUR TIMES DAILY
- **ECHINACEA:** 400 MG FOUR TIMES DAILY
- **CAT'S CLAW:** 2,000 MG FOUR TIMES DAILY
- **QUERCETIN:** 1,000 MG FOUR TIMES DAILY
- **ANDROGRAPHIS:** 600 MG FOUR TIMES DAILY
- **ZHONG GAN LING:** 10 PILLS FOUR TIMES DAILY

or follow the advice of a licensed acupuncturist and Oriental medicine specialist.

Should you become very sick, in addition to the maximum intervention regimen of prescription 3, you'll need to optimize your program to achieve the full potential of natural medicines in order to beat the flu. In addition to increasing dosages and the frequency of how many times you take these medicines, you may also require physician-administered medications. Prescription 4 offers some guidelines to help you choose which ones are best for treating a serious infection.

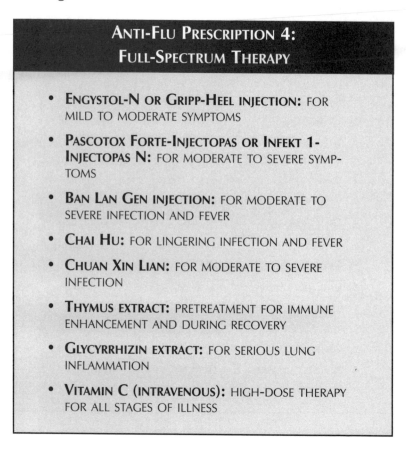

**ANTI-FLU PRESCRIPTION 4:
FULL-SPECTRUM THERAPY**

- **ENGYSTOL-N OR GRIPP-HEEL INJECTION:** FOR MILD TO MODERATE SYMPTOMS

- **PASCOTOX FORTE-INJECTOPAS OR INFEKT 1-INJECTOPAS N:** FOR MODERATE TO SEVERE SYMPTOMS

- **BAN LAN GEN INJECTION:** FOR MODERATE TO SEVERE INFECTION AND FEVER

- **CHAI HU:** FOR LINGERING INFECTION AND FEVER

- **CHUAN XIN LIAN:** FOR MODERATE TO SEVERE INFECTION

- **THYMUS EXTRACT:** PRETREATMENT FOR IMMUNE ENHANCEMENT AND DURING RECOVERY

- **GLYCYRRHIZIN EXTRACT:** FOR SERIOUS LUNG INFLAMMATION

- **VITAMIN C (INTRAVENOUS):** HIGH-DOSE THERAPY FOR ALL STAGES OF ILLNESS

WHEN SHOULD I STOP TAKING NATURAL MEDICINES?

Don't stop taking natural medicines until well after symptoms are gone. For a common cold or ordinary flu, that's about one to two weeks. For a more severe bout of seasonal influenza, continue for three to four weeks. If you are not getting better or have lingering symptoms such as fatigue or coughing, you may have to take natural medications for four to six weeks.

For a highly virulent pandemic flu, I recommend continuing well beyond elimination of symptoms. Take natural medicines for six to eight weeks and up to three months from the onset of infection. It's best not to take chances with something as serious as a pandemic virus.

Should a super flu emerge, it's likely that it will cover the globe in several progressive waves. It may mutate, spawning multiple versions of the same flu, so you could get sick repeatedly until your body has developed natural immunity to fight it off or the virus weakens. If this were the case, you and your family may have to stay on a regime of natural medications for three to six months.

Long-term use of nutritional supplements, if taken in the recommended dosages, poses no overdosing risk. Homeopathic medicines are safe and, as a rule, are only taken to control symptoms or when necessary to treat a condition. Overdosing is not an issue. Immune-enhancing medications are also safe when taken as recommended. The herbs listed in this book are safe and pose little risk of adverse effects; however, they are not intended to be taken for longer than three months without supervision by a healthcare practitioner knowledgeable in their use. Once all symptoms are gone and the risk of repeated infection is over, you can discontinue natural medications.

Complications of influenza can be worse than the flu itself. Among the most perilous is the body's own exaggerated immune response. When severe, it causes high fever, crippling body pain, and weakness. If excessive, it can cause tissue damage that may lead to organ failure and death. Other complications include nerve and muscle damage and even brain injury. Weakness or inflammation of lung tissue as an aftermath of coughing can occur, with symptoms lingering for months. Adverse events from vaccination and drugs are likely to occur in many people.

It's possible that a super flu can cause problems long after the viral infection is over. Therefore it's important to practice effective postinfection care even after symptoms have passed. In the best-case scenario, if you get sick and you treat it early and effectively, you'll recover within two to four weeks without complications. It's possible, however, that after severe influenza, as long as 12 weeks may be required to feel like you're back to normal. If you're not on the way to recovery three weeks after the onset of symptoms, consider taking Anti-Flu Prescription 5.

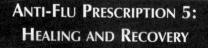

ANTI-FLU PRESCRIPTION 5:
HEALING AND RECOVERY

- **MULTIVITAMIN/MINERAL SUPPLEMENT:** TAKE A BROAD RANGE OF PURE NUTRIENTS WITHOUT IRON IN DIVIDED DOSAGES WITH EACH MEAL.

- **ASTRAGALUS:** FOR LINGERING FATIGUE AND LASSITUDE, TAKE 500 MG OF ASTRAGALUS THREE TIMES DAILY OR MAKE ASTRAGALUS ROOT TEA.

- **GINSENG:** FOR PEOPLE OLDER THAN AGE 50 WITH SEVERE FATIGUE AND LOSS OF MOTIVATION, TAKE 250 MG OF GINSENG EXTRACT DAILY.

- **BUPLEURUM:** FOR LINGERING COUGH AND SHORTNESS OF BREATH, TAKE THE CHINESE HERBAL FORMULA MINOR BUPLEURUM DECOCTION/*XIAO CHAI HU TANG*. THE AVERAGE DOSAGE IS THREE 250 MG CAPSULES THREE TIMES DAILY. IT ALSO COMES IN GRANULE FORM TO BE MADE INTO AN INSTANT HERBAL BEVERAGE. MIX ONE PACKET PER CUP OF HOT WATER AND DRINK 1 CUP THREE TIMES DAILY.

You've come to the end of the book. I hope it has educated you and that you'll look on it as a guide to surviving a pandemic. It is my sincere wish that you will use the natural medicines I discuss to achieve a healthy balance, enhanced viral immunity, and a stronger constitution, and to survive an influenza pandemic.

ACKNOWLEDGMENTS

I am grateful to the many people who have advised, guided, and supported me along the way in writing this book. My foremost thanks go to Sara Sgarlat and Jack Jennings of Hampton Roads Publishing for their unwavering support. Thanks to Judy Goldstein, M.D., Jay S. Cohen, M.D., Minton "Chip" Dobson of Chilsom Labs, Sheldon Saul Hendler, M.D., Ph.D., Jake Paul Fratkin, O.M.D., L.Ac., Alan J. Sault, M.D., Partha Banerjee, M.D., Ye DeBao, Ph.D., Andrei Chugunov, M.D., Ph.D., and Jim Chan, N.D.

RESOURCES

WEBSITES

Centers for Disease Control and Prevention
www.cdc.gov/flu/pandemic

World Health Organization
www.who.int/csr/disease/influenza/pandemic/en

Official U.S. Government Website for Pandemic Flu and Avian
    Influenza
www.pandemicflu.gov/general

Public Health Agency of Canada
www.phac-aspc.gc.ca/influenza/pandemicplan_e.html

Avian Influenza
www.avianinfluenza.org

Enflu
www.enflu.com

Eurosurveillance
www.eurosurveillance.org/em/v03n03/0303-223.asp

FluSTAR System for Reporting and Tracking Flu
www.flustar.com

Humanitarian Early Warning Service
www.hewsweb.org/avian_flu

Rehydration Project
www.rehydrate.org/solutions/homemade.htm

Beating the Flu

BLOGS

Bird Flu
Bird-flu-symptom.info/category/symptoms

Flu Wiki
www.fluwikie.com/index.php?n=Main.HomePage

Global Bird Flu Preparedness Organization
www.vgb.no/3491

H5N1 News and Resources about Avian Flu
Crofsblogs.typepad.com/h5n1

SUPPLIERS

Aethlon Medical
www.aethlonmedical.com

Emerson Ecologics
7 Commerce Drive, Bedford, NH 03110
www.emersonecologics.com

German Society for Thymus Therapy
www.thymus-therapie.org

Heel
P.O. Box 11280, Albuquerque, NM 87192-0280
www.heelusa.com

Mayway Corporation
1338 Mandela Parkway, Oakland, CA 94607
www.mayway.com

Oscillococcinum
www.oscilloinfo.com

PASCOE Naturmedizin
www.pascoe.de

Pure Prescriptions
535 Encinitas Blvd., Suite 118, Encinitas, CA 92024
www.pureprescriptions.com

Viroxx Air Sterilization
www.viroxx.de

Willner Chemists
100 Park Ave., New York, NY 10017
www.willner.com

CENTERS AND ORGANIZATIONS

Alternative Medicine Foundation
P.O. Box 60016, Potomac, MD 20859
www.amfoundation.org

American Academy of Anti-Aging Medicine
1510 W. Montana St., Chicago, IL 60614
www.worldhealth.net

American Association of Integrative Medicine
2750 E. Sunshine, Springfield, MO 65804
www.aaimedicine.com/main.php

American Association of Naturopathic Physicians
8201 Greensboro Dr., Suite 300, McLean, VA 22102
www.naturopathic.org

American Association of Oriental Medicine
433 Front St., Catasauqua, PA 18932
www.aaom.org

American College for Advancement in Medicine
23121 Verdugo Dr., Suite 204, Laguna Hills, CA 92653
www.acam.org

American Osteopathic Association
142 E. Ontario St., Chicago, IL 60611
www.aoa-net.org

British Columbia Naturopathic Association
2238 Pine St., Vancouver, BC V6J 5G4 Canada
www.bcna.ca

National Center for Complementary and Alternative Medicine
P.O. Box 7923, Gaithersburg, MD 20898
www.nccam.nih.gov

Beating the Flu

National Center for Homeopathy
801 N. Fairfax St., Suite 306, Alexandria, VA 22314
www.homeopathic.org

National Institute of Health
9000 Rockville Pike, Bethesda, MD 20892
www.nih.gov

GLOSSARY

ANDROGEN: A hormone associated with masculinizing features.

ANTIBODY: A protein found in the blood that binds with an antigen and that is formed in response to an infection or immunization.

ANTIGEN: A foreign molecule or microbe such as a virus that stimulates antibody formation.

ANTIGENIC DRIFT: The gradual re-assortment of influenza genes over time.

ANTIGENIC SHIFT: The unpredictable and rapid rearrangement of influenza genes resulting in a new virus.

AVASCULAR NECROSIS: A degenerative bone disease that can be caused by overuse of corticosteroid drugs and that results in crippling arthritis and bone loss.

AVIAN INFLUENZA: An infection caused by influenza virus that occurs naturally in birds.

B-CELL: A white blood cell crucial to immune defenses that develops in the bone marrow and is involved in recognition of virus-infected cells.

BIRD FLU: The H5N1 type of avian influenza. A virus.

CYTOKINE: A protein produced by immune cells that influences the immunological behavior and activity of other cells.

CYTOTOXIC T-CELL: A white blood cell that kills virus-infected cells and keeps cancer cells in check.

ENDEMIC: A pattern of disease that commonly occurs in a particular geographic region.

EPIDEMIC: A pattern of disease involving rapid spread and a large number of victims and that occurs over a wide geographical area.

EVIDENCE-BASED MEDICINE: A medical model that uses different levels of scientific research to support the practice of clinical therapies.

Beating the Flu

GANMAO: The Chinese word for seasonal flu and common cold.

GUILLAIN-BARRÉ SYNDROME: A rare crippling nervous system disease marked by severe fatigue.

HEMAGGLUTININ (HA): One of two protein spikes found on the surface of an influenza virus responsible for binding to the cell that is being infected.

HOMEOPATHY: A system of medicine that uses minute dosages of a substance to treat disease and restore homeostasis.

HOMOTOXICOLOGY: A system of medicine that utilizes specialized homeopathic preparations to treat disease by removing toxins from the body's cells and tissues.

IMMUNOGLOBULINS: Immune-enhancing substances found in mother's milk and commercial colostrum.

INFLAMMATION: A localized or systemic event following an injury or infection characterized by redness, swelling, warmth, and pain.

INFLUENZA (FLU): The illness caused by an RNA virus of which there are three types: influenza A, B, and C.

INTERFERON: A group of cytokines involved in communication between immune cells that has particular importance in protection against viral infection.

LYMPHOCYTE: A type of white blood cell involved in immunity and composed of two fundamental groups of cells, T-cells and B-cells.

MATERIA MEDICA: The Latin medical term for a body of therapeutic knowledge about substances used for healing.

NATURAL KILLER CELL: A type of lymphocyte that recognizes and kills cells infected by viruses.

NATUROPATHY: A system of medicine that utilizes a wide variety of natural therapies such as herbal medicine to treat disease and restore health.

NEURAMINIDASE: The mushroom-shaped protein spike found on the surface of the influenza virus involved in promoting the release of new viruses from infected cells.

PANDEMIC: A global epidemic.

PATHOGEN: A disease-causing microorganism.

SEVERE ACUTE RESPIRATORY SYNDROME (SARS): The epidemic characterized by respiratory infection that started in Hong Kong in 2003, caused by a coronavirus that spread from civet cats to people.

SUPER SPREADER: A single sick person infecting countless others, increasing exponentially the transmission of disease.

T-CELL (T LYMPHOCYTE): An immune cell that develops in the thymus gland and helps manage infection.

TRADITIONAL CHINESE MEDICINE (TCM): A system of medicine developed in China that includes acupuncture, herbal medicine, and a variety of other therapies, techniques, and practices to treat disease and restore health by regulating the balance of yin and yang.

VACCINE: A medically prepared microbial antigen used to induce an immune response and provide protection against infection.

VIRON: A single viral particle.

VIRULENCE: The degree or severity of illness an infectious organism is capable of causing.

VIRUS: An intracellular parasitic organism involved in a wide range of diseases.

WEN BING: The Chinese term for febrile epidemic influenza-like respiratory tract disease.

SELECTED BIBLIOGRAPHY

Abel G, JK Czop. "Stimulation of Human Monocyte Beta-Glucan Receptors by Glucan Particles Induces Production of TNF-Alpha and IL-1 Beta." *International Journal of Immunopharmacology* 14 (1992): 1363–73.

Akkerman AE, MM Kuyvenhoven, JC van der Wouden, TJ Verheij. "Determinants of Antibiotic Overprescribing in Respiratory Tract Infections in General Practice." *Journal of Antimicrobial Chemotherapy* 56, no. 5 (2005): 930–6.

———. "Prescribing Antibiotics for Respiratory Tract Infections by GPs: Management and Prescriber Characteristics." *British Journal of General Practice* 55, no. 511 (2005): 114–8.

Allsup SJ, M Gosney, M Regan, et al. "Side Effects of Influenza Vaccination in Healthy Older People: A Randomized Single-Blind Placebo-Controlled Trial." *Gerontology* 47, no. 6 (2001): 311–4.

Atigadda VR, WJ Brouillette, F Duarte, et al. "Hydrophobic Benzoic Acids as Inhibitors of Influenza Neuraminidase." *Bioorganic and Medicinal Chemistry* 7, no. 11 (1999): 2487–97.

Austenaa LM, H Carlsen, A Ertesvag, et al. "Vitamin A Status Significantly Alters Nuclear Factor-Kappa B Activity Assessed by in Vivo Imaging." *Federation of American Societies for Experimental Biology Journal* 18, no. 11 (2004): 1255–7.

Beigel J. "Interpreting Diagnostic Studies in SARS—Defining the Reference." *Clinical Immunology* 113, no. 2 (2004): 117–8.

Beigel JH, J Farrar, AM Han, et al. "Avian Influenza A (H5N1) Infection in Humans." *New England Journal of Medicine* 353, no. 13 (2005): 1374–85.

Berkhoff EG, E de Wit, MM Geelhoed-Mieras, et al. "Functional Constraints of Influenza A Virus Epitopes Limit Escape from Cytotoxic T Lymphocytes." *Journal of Virology* 79, no. 17 (2005): 11239–46.

Beveridge, WIB. *Influenza: The Last Great Plague*. New York: Prodist, 1978.

Blomhoff HK. "Vitamin A Regulates Proliferation and Apoptosis of Human T- and B-Cells." *Biochemical Society Transactions* 32, Pt 6 (2004): 982–4.

Bock K, N Sabin. *The Road to Immunity: How to Survive and Thrive in a Toxic World*. New York: Pocket Books, 1997.

Bone K. "Echinacea: What Makes It Work?" *Alternative Medicine Review* 2, no. 2 (1997): 87–93.

———. "Echinacea: When Should It Be Used?" *Alternative Medicine Review* 2, no. 6 (1997): 451–8.

Boon AC, G de Mutsert, RA Fouchier, et al. "Functional Profile of Human

Influenza Virus-Specific Cytotoxic T Lymphocyte Activity Is Influenced by Interleukin-2 Concentration and Epitope Specificity." *Clinical and Experimental Immunology* 142, no. 1 (2005): 45–52.

Boon AC, E Fringuelli, YM Graus, et al. "Influenza A Virus Specific T-Cell Immunity in Humans during Aging." *Virology* 299, no. 1 (2002): 100–8.

Boon AC, AP Vos, YM Graus, et al. "In Vitro Effect of Bioactive Compounds on Influenza Virus Specific B- and T-Cell Responses." *Scandinavian Journal of Immunology* 55, no. 1 (2002): 24–32.

Brinker, Francis. *Herb Contraindications and Drug Interactions.* Sandy, Ore.: Eclectic Medical Publications, 1998.

Bueving HJ, RM Bernsen, JC de Jongste, et al. "Does Influenza Vaccination Exacerbate Asthma in Children?" *Vaccine* 23, no. 1 (2004): 91–6.

Bueving HJ, JC van der Wouden, MY Berger, S Thomas. "Incidence of Influenza and Associated Illness in Children Aged 0–19 Years: A Systematic Review." *Reviews in Medical Virology* 15, no. 6 (2005): 383–91.

Burger RA, AR Torres, RP Warren, et al. "Echinacea-Induced Cytokine Production by Human Macrophages." *International Journal of Immunopharmacology* 19, no. 7 (1997): 371–9.

Camuesco D, M Comalada, ME Rodriguez-Cabezas, et al. "The Intestinal Anti-Inflammatory Effect of Quercetin Is Associated with an Inhibition in INOS Expression." *British Journal of Pharmacology* 143, no. 7 (2004): 908–18.

Canney S. "Cordyceps Sinensis: Animal, Vegetable, or Both?" *Journal of Chinese Medicine* 80 (February 2006): 40–7.

Carr A, DA Cooper. "Adverse Effects of Antiretroviral Therapy." *Lancet* 356 (2000): 1423–30.

Chan KH, LL Poon, VC Cheng, Y Guan, et al. "Detection of SARS Coronavirus in Patients with Suspected SARS." *Emerging Infectious Diseases* 10, no. 2 (2004): 294–9.

Chan MC, CY Cheung, WH Chui, et al. "Proinflammatory Cytokine Responses Induced by Influenza A (H5N1) Viruses in Primary Human Alveolar and Bronchial Epithelial Cells." *Respiratory Research* 6 (2005): 135.

Chandra RK. "Nutrition and Immunology: From the Clinic to Cellular Biology and Back Again." *Proceedings of the Nutritional Society* 58, no. 3 (1999): 681–3.

———. "Nutrition and the Immune System: An Introduction." *American Journal of Clinical Nutrition* 66 (1997): 460S–63S.

———. "Nutrition, Immunity, and Infection: From Basic Knowledge of Dietary Manipulation of Immune Responses to Practical Application of Ameliorating Suffering and Improving Survival." *Proceedings of the National Academy of Sciences USA* 93 (1996): 14304–7.

Chatterjee P. "Hong Kong Battens Down the Hatches." *Lancet* 366, no. 9503 (2005): 2073–74.

Chen H, G Deng, Z Li, et al. "The Evolution of H5N1 Influenza Viruses in Ducks in Southern China." *Proceedings of the National Academy of Sciences U S A* 101, no. 28 (2004): 10452–7.

Chen H, GJ Smith, SY Zhang, et al. "Avian Flu: H5N1 Virus Outbreak in Migratory Waterfowl." *Nature* 436, no. 7048 (2005): 191–2.

Chen KT, SJ Twu, HL Chang, et al. "SARS in Taiwan: An Overview and Lessons Learned." *International Journal of Infectious Disease* 9, no. 2 (2005): 77–85.

Cheng MH. "Influenza Pandemic Preparedness." *Lancet Infectious Diseases* 5, no. 12 (2005): 740.

Chin PS, E Hoffmann, R Webby, et al. "Molecular Evolution of H6 Influenza Viruses from Poultry in Southeastern China: Prevalence of H6N1 Influenza Viruses Possessing Seven A/Hong Kong/156/97 (H5N1)-Like Genes in Poultry." *Journal of Virology* 76, no. 2 (2002): 507–16.

Choi AM, K Knobil, SL Otterbein, et al. "Oxidant Stress Responses in Influenza Virus Pneumonia: Gene Expression and Transcription Factor Activation." *American Journal of Physiology* 271, no. 3 Pt 1 (1996): L383–91.

Choi YK, TD Nguyen, H Ozaki, et al. "Studies of H5N1 Influenza Virus Infection of Pigs by Using Viruses Isolated in Vietnam and Thailand in 2004." *Journal of Virology* 79, no. 16 (2005): 10821–5.

Choi YK, SH Seo, JA Kim, et al. "Avian Influenza Viruses in Korean Live Poultry Markets and Their Pathogenic Potential." *Virology* 332, no. 2 (2005): 529–37.

Chokephaibulkit K, M Uiprasertkul, P Puthavathana, et al. "A Child with Avian Influenza A (H5N1) Infection." *Pediatric Infectious Disease Journal* 24, no. 2 (2005): 162–6.

Collier, Leslie, and John Oxford. *Human Virology.* New York: Oxford University Press, 2000.

Comalada M, D Camuesco, S Sierra, et al. "In Vivo Quercitrin Anti-Inflammatory Effect Involves Release of Quercetin, Which Inhibits Inflammation through Down-Regulation of the NF-Kappa B Pathway." *European Journal of Immunology* 35, no. 2 (2005): 584–92.

Crawford, Dorothy H. *The Invisible Enemy: A Natural History of Viruses.* New York: Oxford University Press, 2000.

Cui D, Z Moldoveanu, CB Stephensen. "High-Level Dietary Vitamin A Enhances T-Helper Type 2 Cytokine Production and Secretory Immunoglobulin A Response to Influenza A Virus Infection in Balb/C Mice." *Journal of Nutrition* 130, no. 5 (2000): 1132–9.

Currier NL, SC Miller. "Echinacea Purpurea and Melatonin Augment Natural-Killer Cells in Leukemic Mice and Prolong Life Span." *Journal of Alternative and Complementary Medicine* 7, no. 3 (2001): 241–51.

Damoiseaux R, JC van der Wouden, H Bueving. "Influenza Vaccination Effectiveness Is Not Proven in Younger Individuals at Risk." *Archives of Internal Medicine* 165, no. 16 (2005): 1921–2; author reply 1922.

De Flora S, C Grassi, L Carati. "Attenuation of Influenza-Like Symptomatology and Improvement of Cell-Mediated Immunity with Long-Term N-Acetylcysteine Treatment." *European Respiratory Journal* 10, no. 7 (1997): 1535–41.

Desselberger U, K Nakajima, P Alfino, et al. "Biochemical Evidence That 'New' Influenza Virus Strains in Nature May Arise by Recombination (Reassortment)." *Proceedings of the National Academy of Sciences U S A* 75, no. 7 (1978): 3341–5.

Diamond, Jared. *Guns, Germs, and Steel.* New York: WW Norton, 1997.

Diluzio NR. "Immunopharmacology of Glucan: A Broad-Spectrum Enhancer of Host Defense Mechanisms." *Trends in Pharmacology* 4 (1983): 433–47.

Donnelly LE, R Newton, GE Kennedy, et al. "Anti-Inflammatory Effects of Resveratrol in Lung Epithelial Cells: Molecular Mechanisms." *American Journal of Physiology, Lung Cellular and Molecular Physiology* 287, no. 4 (2004): L774–83.

Dowell SF. "Seasonal Variation in Host Susceptibility and Cycles of Certain Infectious Diseases." *Emerging Infectious Diseases* 7, no. 3 (2001): 369–74.

Dowell SF, MS Ho. "Seasonality of Infectious Diseases and Severe Acute Respiratory Syndrome—What We Don't Know Can Hurt Us." *Lancet Infectious Diseases* 4, no. 11 (2004): 704–8.

Dowell SF, B Schwartz, WR Phillips. "Appropriate Use of Antibiotics for URIs in Children: Part I. Otitis Media and Acute Sinusitis. The Pediatric URI Consensus Team." *American Family Physician* 58, no. 5 (1998): 1113–8, 1123.

Dowell SF, JM Simmerman, DD Erdman, et al. "Severe Acute Respiratory Syndrome Coronavirus on Hospital Surfaces." *Clinical Infectious Diseases* 39, no. 5 (2004): 652–7.

Dreffier C, F Ramisse, JM Alonso. "Immunoprophylaxis of Respiratory Infections." *Medical Science (Paris)* 20, no. 11 (2004): 999–1003.

Eccles R. "Understanding the Symptoms of the Common Cold and Influenza." *Lancet Infectious Diseases* 5, no. 11 (2005): 718–25.

Engedal N, A Ertesvag, HK Blomhoff. "Survival of Activated Human T Lymphocytes Is Promoted by Retinoic Acid via Induction of IL-2." *International Immunology* 16, no. 3 (2004): 443–53.

Epstein SL, TM Tumpey, JA Misplon, et al. "DNA Vaccine Expressing Conserved Influenza Virus Proteins Protective against H5N1 Challenge Infection in Mice." *Emerging Infectious Diseases* 8, no. 8 (2002): 796–801.

Ertesvag A, N Engedal, S Naderi, HK Blomhoff. "Retinoic Acid Stimulates the Cell Cycle Machinery in Normal T-Cells: Involvement of Retinoic Acid Receptor-Mediated Il-2 Secretion." *Journal of Immunology* 169, no. 10 (2002): 5555–63.

Ewald, Paul W. *Evolution of Infectious Disease*. New York: Oxford University Press, 1994.

Fettner, Ann Giudici. *Viruses: Agents of Change*. New York: McGraw-Hill, 1990.

Fleming, Thomas, ed. *PDR for Herbal Medicines*. Montvale, N.J.: Medical Economics, 1998.

Flint, SJ, LW Enquist, RM Krug, et al. *Principles of Virology, Molecular Biology, Pathogenesis, and Control*. Washington, D.C.: ASM Press, 2000.

Franks TJ, PY Chong, P Chui, et al. "Lung Pathology of Severe Acute Respiratory Syndrome (SARS): A Study of Eight Autopsy Cases from Singapore." *Human Pathology* 34, no. 8 (2003): 743–8.

Gabriel G, B Dauber, T Wolff, et al. "The Viral Polymerase Mediates Adaptation of an Avian Influenza Virus to a Mammalian Host." *Proceedings of the National Academy of Sciences U S A* 102, no. 51 (2005): 18590–5.

Galan P, P Preziosi, AL Monget, et al. "Effects of Trace Element and/or Vitamin Supplementation on Vitamin and Mineral Status, Free Radical Metabolism, and Immunological Markers in Elderly Long-Term-Hospitalized Subjects. Geriatric Network MIN. VIT. AOX." *International Journal for Vitamin and Nutrition Research* 67, no. 6 (1997): 450–60.

Gambaryan AS, AB Tuzikov, AA Chinarev, et al. "Polymeric Inhibitor of Influenza Virus Attachment Protects Mice from Experimental Influenza Infection." *Antiviral Research* 55, no. 1 (2002): 201–5.

Gambaryan AS, AB Tuzikov, GV Pazynina, et al. "H5N1 Chicken Influenza Viruses Display a High Binding Affinity for Neu5Acalpha2-3Galbeta1-4(6-HSO3)GlcNAc-Containing Receptors." *Virology* 326, no. 2 (2004): 310–6.

Garman E, G Laver. "Controlling Influenza by Inhibiting the Virus's Neuraminidase." *Current Drug Targets* 5, no. 2 (2004): 119–36.

Geiss GK, M Salvatore, TM Tumpey, et al. "Cellular Transcriptional Profiling in Influenza A Virus-Infected Lung Epithelial Cells: The Role of the Nonstructural NS1 Protein in the Evasion of the Host Innate Defense and Its Potential Contribution to Pandemic Influenza." *Proceedings of the National Academy of Sciences U S A* 99, no. 16 (2002): 10736–41.

Ghedin E, NA Sengamalay, M Shumway, et al. "Large-Scale Sequencing of Human Influenza Reveals the Dynamic Nature of Viral Genome Evolution." *Nature* 437, no. 7062 (2005): 1162–6.

Ghezzi P, D Ungheri. "Synergistic Combination of N-Acetylcysteine and Ribavirin to Protect from Lethal Influenza Viral Infection in a Mouse Model." *International Journal of Immunopathology and Pharmacology* 17, no. 1 (2004): 99–102.

Giansanti F, P Rossi, MT Massucci, et al. "Antiviral Activity of Ovotransferrin Discloses an Evolutionary Strategy for the Defensive Activities of Lactorferrin." *Biochemistry and Cell Biology* 80, no. 1 (2002): 125–30.

Girodon F, MC Boutron-Ruault, P Galan, S Hercberg. "Vitamin Supplementation in Elderly Persons." *Journal of the American Medical Association* 289, no. 2 (2003): 173–4; author reply 174.

Girodon F, P Galan, AL Monget, et al. "Impact of Trace Elements and Vitamin Supplementation on Immunity and Infections in Institutionalized Elderly Patients: A Randomized Controlled Trial. MIN. VIT. AOX. Geriatric Network." *Archives of Internal Medicine* 159, no. 7 (1999): 748–54.

Glaser L, J Stevens, D Zamarin, et al. "A Single Amino Acid Substitution in 1918 Influenza Virus Hemagglutinin Changes Receptor Binding Specificity." *Journal of Virology* 79, no. 17 (2005): 11533–6.

Govorkova EA, IA Leneva, OG Goloubeva, et al. "Comparison of Efficacies of RWJ-270201, Zanamivir, and Oseltamivir against H5N1, H9N2, and Other Avian Influenza Viruses." *Antimicrobial Agents and Chemotherapy* 45, no. 10 (2001): 2723–32.

Govorkova EA, JE Rehg, S Krauss, et al. "Lethality to Ferrets of H5N1 Influenza Viruses Isolated from Humans and Poultry in 2004." *Journal of Virology* 79, no. 4 (2005): 2191–8.

Guan Y, LL Poon, CY Cheung, et al. "H5N1 Influenza: A Protean Pandemic Threat." *Proceedings of the National Academy of Sciences U S A* 101, no. 21 (2004): 8156–61.

Beating the Flu

Gubareva LV, L Kaiser, MN Matrosovich, et al. "Selection of Influenza Virus Mutants in Experimentally Infected Volunteers Treated with Oseltamivir." *Journal of Infectious Diseases* 183, no. 4 (2001): 523–31.

Hagen E, AM Myhre, S Smeland, et al. "Uptake of Vitamin A in Macrophages from Physiologic Transport Proteins: Role of Retinol-Binding Protein and Chylomicron Remnants." *Journal of Nutritional Biochemistry* 10, no. 6 (1999): 345–52.

Hanekom WA, R Yogev, LM Heald, et al. "Effect of Vitamin A Therapy on Serologic Responses and Viral Load Changes after Influenza Vaccination in Children Infected with the Human Immunodeficiency Virus." *Journal of Pediatrics* 136, no. 4 (2000): 550–2.

Hawkins MG, BM Crossley, A Osofsky, et al. "Avian Influenza A Virus Subtype H5N2 in a Red-Lored Amazon Parrot." *Journal of the American Veterinary Medical Association* 228, no. 2 (2006): 236–41.

Hayden F, A Klimov, M Tashiro, et al. "Neuraminidase Inhibitor Susceptibility Network Position Statement: Antiviral Resistance in Influenza A/H5N1 Viruses." *Antiviral Therapy* 10, no. 8 (2005): 873–7.

Hernandez E, F Ramisse, P Gros, J Cavallo. "Super-Infection by Bacillus Thuringiensis H34 or 3a3b Can Lead to Death in Mice Infected with the Influenza A Virus." *FEMS Immunology and Medical Microbiology* 29, no. 3 (2000): 177–81.

Hoelscher MA, S Garg, DS Bangari. "Development of Adenoviral-Vector-Based Pandemic Influenza Vaccine against Antigenically Distinct Human H5N1 Strains in Mice." *Lancet* 376, no. 9509 (2006): 475–81.

Hoffmann E, AS Lipatov, RJ Webby, et al. "Role of Specific Hemagglutinin Amino Acids in the Immunogenicity and Protection of H5N1 Influenza Virus Vaccines." *Proceedings of the National Academy of Sciences U S A* 102, no. 36 (2005): 12915–20.

Hoffmann E, J Stech, I Leneva, et al. "Characterization of the Influenza A Virus Gene Pool in Avian Species in Southern China: Was H6N1 a Derivative or a Precursor of H5N1?" *Journal of Virology* 74, no. 14 (2000): 6309–15.

Holmes EC, JK Taubenberger, BT Grenfell. "Heading Off an Influenza Pandemic." *Science* 309, no. 5737 (2005): 989.

Hulse-Post DJ, KM Sturm-Ramirez, J Humberd, et al. "Role of Domestic Ducks in the Propagation and Biological Evolution of Highly Pathogenic H5N1 Influenza Viruses in Asia." *Proceedings of the National Academy of Sciences USA* 102, no. 30 (2005): 10682–7.

Ilyushina NA, EA Govorkova, RG Webster. "Detection of Amantadine-Resistant Variants among Avian Influenza Viruses Isolated in North America and Asia." *Virology* 341, no. 1 (2005): 102–6.

Jefferson T, V Demicheli, D Rivetti, et al. "Antivirals for Influenza in Healthy Adults: Systematic Review." *Lancet* 367, no. 9507 (2006): 303–13.

Judd AK, A Sanchez, DJ Bucher, et al. "In Vivo Anti-Influenza Virus Activity of a Zinc Finger Peptide." *Antimicrobial Agents and Chemotherapy* 41, no. 3 (1997): 687–v92.

Kash JC, CF Basler, A Garcia-Sastre, et al. "Global Host Immune Response:

Pathogenesis and Transcriptional Profiling of Type A Influenza Viruses Expressing the Hemagglutinin and Neuraminidase Genes from the 1918 Pandemic Virus." *Journal of Virology* 78, no. 17 (2004): 9499–511.

Katz JM, J Plowden, M Renshaw-Hoelscher, et al. "Immunity to Influenza: The Challenges of Protecting an Aging Population." *Immunological Research* 29, no. 1–3 (2004): 113–24.

Kim H, H Kong, B Choi, et al. "Metabolic and Pharmacological Properties of Rutin, a Dietary Quercetin Glycoside, for Treatment of Inflammatory Bowel Disease." *Pharmaceutical Research* 22, no. 9 (2005): 1499–509.

Klaesson S, O Ringden, L Markling, et al. "Immune Modulatory Effects of Immunoglobulins on Cell-Mediated Immune Responses in Vitro." *Scandinavian Journal of Immunology* 38, no. 5 (1993): 477–84.

Knobil K, AM Choi, GW Weigand, DB Jacoby. "Role of Oxidants in Influenza Virus-Induced Gene Expression." *American Journal of Physiology* 274, no. 1, Pt 1 (1998): L134–42.

Koren G, S King, S Knowles, E Phillips. "Ribavirin in the Treatment of SARS: A New Trick for an Old Drug?" *Canadian Medical Association Journal* 168, no. 10 (2003): 1289–92.

Krauss S, D Walker, SP Pryor, et al. "Influenza A Viruses of Migrating Wild Aquatic Birds in North America." *Vector Borne Zoonotic Diseases* 4, no. 3 (2004): 177–89.

Ksiazek TG, D Erdman, CS Goldsmith, et al. "A Novel Coronavirus Associated with Severe Acute Respiratory Syndrome." *New England Journal of Medicine* 348, no. 20 (2003): 1953–66.

Kummer C. "Spring Chickens." *Atlantic Monthly* (April 2006): 127–32.

Lau TF, PC Leung, ELY Wong, et al. "Using Herbal Medicine as a Means of Prevention Experience during SARS Crisis." *American Journal of Chinese Medicine* 33, no. 3 (2005): 345–56.

Laver G. "Influenza Drug Could Abort a Pandemic." *Nature* 434, no. 7035 (2005): 821.

Laver G, E Garman. "Pandemic Influenza: Its Origin and Control." *Microbes and Infection* 4, no. 13 (2002): 1309–16.

———. "Virology. The Origin and Control of Pandemic Influenza." *Science* 293, no. 5536 (2001): 1776–7.

Le QM, M Kiso, K Someya, et al. "Avian Flu: Isolation of Drug-Resistant H5N1 Virus." *Nature* 437, no. 7062 (2005): 1108.

Lee VJ, KH Phua, MI Chenm, et al. "Economics of Neuraminidase Inhibitor Stockpiling for Pandemic Influenza, Singapore." *Emerging Infectious Diseases* 12, no. 1 (2006): 95–102.

Leneva IA, O Goloubeva, RJ Fenton, et al. "Efficacy of Zanamivir against Avian Influenza A Viruses That Possess Genes Encoding H5N1 Internal Proteins and Are Pathogenic in Mammals." *Antimicrobial Agents and Chemotherapy* 45, no. 4 (2001): 1216–24.

Li KS, Y Guan, J Wang, et al. "Genesis of a Highly Pathogenic and Potentially Pandemic H5N1 Influenza Virus in Eastern Asia." *Nature* 430, no. 6996 (2004): 209–13.

Beating the Flu

Li Z, H Chen, P Jiao, et al. "Molecular Basis of Replication of Duck H5N1 Influenza Viruses in a Mammalian Mouse Model." *Journal of Virology* 79, no. 18 (2005): 12058–64.

Lin YP, M Shaw, V Gregory, et al. "Avian-to-Human Transmission of H9N2 Subtype Influenza A Viruses: Relationship between H9N2 and H5N1 Human Isolates." *Proceedings of the National Academy of Sciences U S A* 97, no. 17 (2000): 9654–8.

Lipatov AC, IuA Smirnov, NV Kaverin, RG Webster. "[Evolution of Avian Influenza Viruses H5N1 (1997–2004) in Southern and South-Eastern Asia]." *Voprosy Virusologii* 50, no. 4 (2005): 11–7.

Lipatov AS, EA Govorkova, RJ Webby, et al. "Influenza: Emergence and Control." *Journal of Virology* 78, no. 17 (2004): 8951–9.

Liu J, X Li, Y Yue, et al. "The Inhibitory Effect of Quercetin on IL-6 Production by Lps-Stimulated Neutrophils." *Cellular and Molecular Immunology* 2, no. 6 (2005): 455–60.

Liu M, Y Guan, M Peiris, et al. "The Quest of Influenza A Viruses for New Hosts." *Avian Diseases* 47, no. 3 Suppl (2003): 849–56.

Liu X, M Zhang, L He, et al. "Chinese Herbs Combined with Western Medicine for Severe Acute Respiratory Syndrome (SARS)." *Cochrane Database Systematic Reviews*, no. 1 (2006): CD004882.

Lu X, M Renshaw, TM Tumpey, et al. "Immunity to Influenza A H9N2 Viruses Induced by Infection and Vaccination." *Journal of Virology* 75, no. 10 (2001): 4896–901.

Macias A, S Arce, J Leon, et al. "Novel Cross-Reactive Anti-Idiotype Antibodies with Properties Close to the Human Intravenous Immunoglobulin (IVIg)." *Hybridoma* 18, no. 3 (1999): 263–72.

Magnussen CR, RG Douglas Jr., RF Betts, et al. "Double-Blind Evaluation of Oral Ribavirin (Virazole) in Experimental Influenza A Virus Infection in Volunteers." *Antimicrobial Agents and Chemotherapy* 12, no. 4 (1977): 498–502.

Maines TR, XH Lu, SM Erb, et al. "Avian Influenza (H5N1) Viruses Isolated from Humans in Asia in 2004 Exhibit Increased Virulence in Mammals." *Journal of Virology* 79, no. 18 (2005): 11788–800.

Matrosovich MN, S Krauss, RG Webster. "H9N2 Influenza A Viruses from Poultry in Asia Have Human Virus-Like Receptor Specificity." *Virology* 281, no. 2 (2001): 156–62.

Matrosovich MN, TY Matrosovich, T Gray, et al. "Human and Avian Influenza Viruses Target Different Cell Types in Cultures of Human Airway Epithelium." *Proceedings of the National Academy of Sciences U S A* 101, no. 13 (2004): 4620–4.

Mermel LA. "Pandemic Avian Influenza." *Lancet Infectious Diseases* 5, no. 11 (2005): 666–67.

Mimas FM. "Avian Influenza and UV-B Blocked by Biomass Smoke." *Environmental Health Perspectives* 113, no. 12 (2005): 806–07.

Muthian G, JJ Bright. "Quercetin, a Flavonoid Phytoestrogen, Ameliorates Experimental Allergic Encephalomyelitis by Blocking IL-12 Signaling through JAK-STAT Pathway in T Lymphocyte." *Journal of Clinical Immunology* 24, no. 5 (2004): 542–52.

Nair MP, C Kandaswami, S Mahajan, et al. "The Flavonoid Quercetin Differentially Regulates Th-1 (INFgamma) and Th-2 (IL4) Cytokine Gene Expression by Normal Peripheral Blood Mononuclear Cells." *Biochimica Biophysica Acta* 1593, no. 1 (2002): 29–36.

Nair MP, S Mahajan, JL Reynolds, et al. "The Flavonoid Quercetin Inhibits Proinflammatory Cytokine (Tumor Necrosis Factor Alpha) Gene Expression in Normal Peripheral Blood Mononuclear Cells via Modulation of the NF-Kappa Beta System." *Clinical and Vaccine Immunology* 13, no. 3 (2006): 319–28.

Nicholls JM, LL Poon, KC Lee, et al. "Lung Pathology of Fatal Severe Acute Respiratory Syndrome." *Lancet* 361, no. 9371 (2003): 1773–8.

Olsen SJ, Y Laosiritaworn, S Pattanasin, et al. "Poultry-Handling Practices during Avian Influenza Outbreak, Thailand." *Emerging Infectious Diseases* 11, no. 10 (2005): 1601–3.

Olsen SJ, K Ungchusak, L Sovann, et al. "Family Clustering of Avian Influenza A (H5N1)." *Emerging Infectious Diseases* 11, no. 11 (2005): 1799–801.

Oxford JS, Balasingam, R Lambkin. "A New Millennium Conundrum: How to Use a Powerful Class of Influenza Anti-Neuraminidase Drugs (NAIS) in the Community." *Journal of Antimicrobial Chemotherapy* 53, no. 2 (2004): 133–6.

Oxford JS, S Balasingam, C Chan, et al. "New Antiviral Drugs, Vaccines, and Classic Public Health Interventions against SARS Coronavirus." *Antiviral Chemistry & Chemotherapy* 16, no. 1 (2005): 13–21.

Oxford JS, S Bossuyt, S Balasingam, et al. "Treatment of Epidemic and Pandemic Influenza with Neuraminidase and M2 Proton Channel Inhibitors." *Clinical Microbiology and Infection* 9, no. 1 (2003): 1–14.

Oxford JS, R Lambkin, I Gibb, et al. "A Throat Lozenge Containing Amyl Meta Cresol and Dichlorobenzyl Alcohol Has a Direct Virucidal Effect on Respiratory Syncytial Virus, Influenza A, and SARS-COV." *Antiviral Chemistry & Chemotherapy* 16, no. 2 (2005): 129–34.

Palese P, TM Tumpey, A Garcia-Sastre. "What Can We Learn from Reconstructing the Extinct 1918 Pandemic Influenza Virus?" *Immunity* 24, no. 2 (2006): 121–4.

Peat, FD "The Saving of Planet Gaia." *New Scientist* (March 15, 2006): 48–49.

Phua KL, LK Lee. "Meeting the Challenge of Epidemic Infectious Disease Outbreaks: An Agenda for Research." *Journal of Public Health Policy* 26, no. 1 (2005): 122–32.

Poom PMK, CK Wong, KP Fung, et al. "Immunomodulatory Effects of a Traditional Chinese Medicine with Potential Antiviral Activity: A Self-Control Study." *American Journal of Chinese Medicine* 34, no. 1 (2006): 13–21.

Poon LL, Y Guan, JM Nicholls, et al. "The Aetiology, Origins, and Diagnosis of Severe Acute Respiratory Syndrome." *Lancet Infectious Disease* 4, no. 11 (2004): 663–71.

Poon LL, CS Leung, KH Chan, et al. "Recurrent Mutations Associated with Isolation and Passage of SARS Coronavirus in Cells from Non-Human Primates." *Journal of Medical Virology* 76, no. 4 (2005): 435–40.

Provinciali M, A Montenovo, G Di Stefano, et al. "Effect of Zinc or Zinc Plus Arginine Supplementation on Antibody Titre and Lymphocyte Subsets after

Influenza Vaccination in Elderly Subjects: A Randomized Controlled Trial." *Age and Ageing* 27, no. 6 (1998): 715–22.

Ramisse F, FX Deramoudt, M Szatanik, et al. "Effective Prophylaxis of Influenza A Virus Pneumonia in Mice by Topical Passive Immunotherapy with Polyvalent Human Immunoglobulins or F(Ab')2 Fragments." *Clinical and Experimental Immunology* 111, no. 3 (1998): 583–7.

Ritvo P, K Wilson, D Willms. "Vaccines in the Public Eye." *Nature Medicine* 11, no. 4 (2005): S20–4.

Russell CJ, RG Webster. "The Genesis of a Pandemic Influenza Virus." *Cell* 123, no. 3 (2005): 368–71.

Salomon R, J Franks, EA Govorkova, et al. "The Polymerase Complex Genes Contribute to the High Virulence of the Human H5N1 Influenza Virus Isolate A/Vietnam/1203/04." *Journal of Experimental Medicine* 203, no. 3 (2006): 689–97.

Sarkar J, NN Gangopadhyay, Z Moldoveanu, et al. "Vitamin A Is Required for Regulation of Polymeric Immunoglobulin Receptor (PIGR) Expression by Interleukin-4 and Interferon-Gamma in a Human Intestinal Epithelial Cell Line." *Journal of Nutrition* 128, no. 7 (1998): 1063–9.

Seo SH, E Hoffmann, RG Webster. "The NS1 Gene of H5N1 Influenza Viruses Circumvents the Host Antiviral Cytokine Responses." *Virus Research* 103, no. 1–2 (2004): 107–13.

Shinya K, M Ebina, S Yamada, et al. "Avian Flu: Influenza Virus Receptors in the Human Airway." *Nature* 440, no. 7083 (2006): 435–6.

Stephensen CB. "Commentary: A Hypothesis Concerning Vitamin A Supplementation, Vaccines, and Childhood Mortality." *International Journal of Epidemiology* 32, no. 5 (2003): 828–9.

———. "Examining the Effect of a Nutrition Intervention on Immune Function in Healthy Humans: What Do We Mean by Immune Function and Who Is Really Healthy Anyway?" *American Journal of Clinical Nutrition* 74, no. 5 (2001): 565–6.

———. "Vitamin A, Infection, and Immune Function." *Annual Review of Nutrition* 21 (2001): 167–92.

Stephensen CB, LM Franchi, H Hernandez, et al. "Assessment of Vitamin A Status with the Relative-Dose-Response Test in Peruvian Children Recovering from Pneumonia." *American Journal of Clinical Nutrition* 76, no. 6 (2002): 1351–7.

Stephensen CB, X Jiang, T Freytag. "Vitamin A Deficiency Increases the In Vivo Development of IL-10-Positive Th2 Cells and Decreases Development of Th1 Cells in Mice." *Journal of Nutrition* 134, no. 10 (2004): 2660–6.

Stephensen CB, DS Kelley. "The Innate Immune System: Friend and Foe." *American Journal of Clinical Nutrition* 83, no. 2 (2006): 187–8.

Stephensen CB, R Rasooly, X Jiang, et al. "Vitamin A Enhances In Vitro Th2 Development via Retinoid X Receptor Pathway." *Journal of Immunology* 168, no. 9 (2002): 4495–503.

Stevens J, O Blixt, TM Tumpey, et al. "Structure and Receptor Specificity of the Hemagglutinin from an H5N1 Influenza Virus." *Science* 312, no. 5772 (2006):

404–10.

Sturm-Ramirez KM, T Ellis, B Bousfield, et al. "Reemerging H5N1 Influenza Viruses in Hong Kong in 2002 Are Highly Pathogenic to Ducks." *Journal of Virology* 78, no. 9 (2004): 4892–901.

Sturm-Ramirez KM, DJ Hulse-Post, EA Govorkova, et al. "Are Ducks Contributing to the Endemicity of Highly Pathogenic H5N1 Influenza Virus in Asia?" *Journal of Virology* 79, no. 17 (2005): 11269–79.

Taubenberger JK. "The Virulence of the 1918 Pandemic Influenza Virus: Unraveling the Enigma." *Archives of Virology. Supplementum* no. 19 (2005): 101–15.

Taubenberger JK, DM Morens. "1918 Influenza: The Mother of All Pandemics." *Emerging Infectious Diseases* 12, no. 1 (2006): 15–22.

Taubenberger JK, AH Reid, TG Fanning. "Capturing a Killer Flu Virus." *Scientific American* 292, no. 1 (2005): 48–57.

Taubenberger JK, AH Reid, RM Lourens, et al. "Characterization of the 1918 Influenza Virus Polymerase Genes." *Nature* 437, no. 7060 (2005): 889–93.

Thomas PG, R Keating, DJ Hulse-Post, PC Doherty. "Cell-Mediated Protection in Influenza Infection." *Emerging Infectious Diseases* 12, no. 1 (2006): 48–54.

Tumpey TM, CF Basler, PV Aguilar, et al. "Characterization of the Reconstructed 1918 Spanish Influenza Pandemic Virus." *Science* 310, no. 5745 (2005): 77–80.

Tumpey TM, A Garcia-Sastre, A Mikulasova, et al. "Existing Antivirals Are Effective against Influenza Viruses with Genes from the 1918 Pandemic Virus." *Proceedings of the National Academy of Sciences U S A* 99, no. 21 (2002): 13849–54.

Tumpey TM, A Garcia-Sastre, JK Taubenberger, et al. "Pathogenicity and Immunogenicity of Influenza Viruses with Genes from the 1918 Pandemic Virus." *Proceedings of the National Academy of Sciences U S A* 101, no. 9 (2004): 3166–71.

———. A Garcia-Sastre, JK Taubenberger, et al. "Pathogenicity of Influenza Viruses with Genes from the 1918 Pandemic Virus: Functional Roles of Alveolar Macrophages and Neutrophils in Limiting Virus Replication and Mortality in Mice." *Journal of Virology* 79, no. 23 (2005): 14933–44.

Turk S, S Bozfakioglu, ST Ecder, et al. "Effects of Zinc Supplementation on the Immune System and on Antibody Response to Multivalent Influenza Vaccine in Hemodialysis Patients." *International Journal of Artificial Organs* 21, no. 5 (1998): 274–8.

Ungchusak K, P Auewarakul, SF Dowell, et al. "Probable Person-to-Person Transmission of Avian Influenza A (H5N1)." *New England Journal of Medicine* 352, no. 4 (2005): 333–40.

Van der Wouden JC, HJ Bueving, P Poole. "Preventing Influenza: An Overview of Systematic Reviews." *Respiratory Medicine* 99, no. 11 (2005): 1341–9.

Van der Wouden JC, M Monteny, MY Berger. "C-Reactive Protein Values in Viral Respiratory Infections." *British Journal of General Practice* 55, no. 510 (2005): 55.

Vickers A, C Smith. "Homoeopathic Oscillococcinum for Preventing and Treating Influenza and Influenza-Like Syndromes." *Cochrane Database Systematic Reviews*, no. 1 (2004): CD001957.

Villamor E, WW Fawzi. "Effects of Vitamin A Supplementation on Immune

Responses and Correlation with Clinical Outcomes." *Clinical Microbiology Reviews* 18, no. 3 (2005): 446–64.

Visseren FL, JJ Bouwman, KP Bouter, et al. "Procoagulant Activity of Endothelial Cells after Infection with Respiratory Viruses." *Thrombosis and Haemostasis* 84, no. 2 (2000): 319–24.

Visseren FL, MS Verkerk, KP Bouter, et al. "Interleukin-6 Production by Endothelial Cells after Infection with Influenza Virus and Cytomegalovirus." *Journal of Laboratory and Clinical Medicine* 134, no. 6 (1999): 623–30.

Visseren FL, MS Verkerk, T van der Bruggen, et al. "Iron Chelation and Hydroxyl Radical Scavenging Reduce the Inflammatory Response of Endothelial Cells after Infection with Chlamydia Pneumoniae or Influenza A." *European Journal of Clinical Investigation* 32, Suppl 1 (2002): 84–90.

Webby RJ, DR Perez, JS Coleman, et al. "Responsiveness to a Pandemic Alert: Use of Reverse Genetics for Rapid Development of Influenza Vaccines." *Lancet* 363, no. 9415 (2004): 1099–103.

Webby RJ, RG Webster. "Are We Ready for Pandemic Influenza?" *Science* 302, no. 5650 (2003): 1519–22.

Webster R, D Hulse. "Controlling Avian Flu at the Source." *Nature* 435, no. 7041 (2005): 415–6.

Webster RG, Y Guan, L Poon, et al. "The Spread of the H5N1 Bird Flu Epidemic in Asia in 2004." *Archives of Virology. Supplementum*, no. 19 (2005): 117–29.

Webster RG, M Peiris, H Chen, Y Guan. "H5N1 Outbreaks and Enzootic Influenza." *Emerging Infectious Diseases* 12, no. 1 (2006): 3–8.

Widjaja L, SL Krauss, RJ Webby, et al. "Matrix Gene of Influenza A Viruses Isolated from Wild Aquatic Birds: Ecology and Emergence of Influenza A Viruses." *Journal of Virology* 78, no. 16 (2004): 8771–9.

Yen HL, LM Herlocher, E Hoffmann, et al. "Neuraminidase Inhibitor-Resistant Influenza Viruses May Differ Substantially in Fitness and Transmissibility." *Antimicrobial Agents and Chemotherapy* 49, no. 10 (2005): 4075–84.

Zhang MM, XM Liu, L He. "Effect of Integrated Traditional Chinese and Western Medicine on SARS: A Review of Clinical Evidence." *World Journal of Gastroenterology* 10, no. 23 (2004): 3500–5.

Zheng B, ML He, KL Wong, et al. "Potent Inhibition of SARS-Associated Coronavirus (SCOV) Infection and Replication by Type I Interferons (IFN-Alpha/Beta) but Not by Type II Interferon (IFN-Gamma)." *Journal of Interferon and Cytokine Research* 24, no. 7 (2004): 388–90.

Index

Beating the Flu

Beating the Flu

Beating the Flu

About the Author

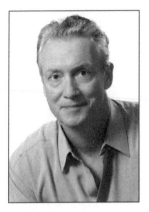

J. E. Williams, O.M.D. is a doctor of Oriental medicine and a fellow of the American Association of Integrative Medicine. He is the academic dean of the East West College of Natural Medicine in Sarasota on the Gulf Coast of Florida. He has served as a professional advisor for national health companies, medical groups, and hospitals including the world famous Scripps Health in La Jolla, California. He travels and lectures extensively on natural therapies and integrative medicine, and is widely published in his field of natural medicine and is the author of *Prolonging Health, Viral Immunity*, and a book on Peruvian shamanism, *The Andean Codex*. For more information on his work and how to live a long healthy life, visit www.doctorwillams.net.

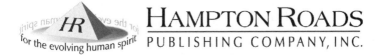

HAMPTON ROADS
PUBLISHING COMPANY, INC.

Thank you for reading Beating the Flu. Hampton Roads is proud to publish an extensive array of books on the topics discussed in Beating the Flu, topics such as viral disease, health, the immune system, and more. Please take a look at the following selection or visit us anytime on the web: www.hrpub.com.

Viral Immunity
A 10-Step Plan to Enhance Your Immunity against Viral Disease Using Natural Medicines
J. E. Williams, O.M.D.

This exceptional health resource sheds light on a host of emerging viral threats from West Nile and Hepatitis to Chronic Fatigue and more, then calmly tells you exactly what you need to know and do to enhance your immunity and prevent, treat, and manage viral conditions.

Paperback • 496 pages • ISBN 1-57174-265-4 • $19.95

Prolonging Health
Mastering the 10 Factors of Longevity
J. E. Williams, O.M.D.

Based on the latest medical findings, Dr. Williams presents a practical, 10-point plan to regain and sustain your health as you age by understanding and changing the ten major causes of aging. He shows how to strengthen your heart, revitalize your brain, rebalance your hormones, repair your DNA, and more.

Paperback • 464 pages • ISBN 1-57174-338-3 • $17.95

Hampton Roads Publishing Company

. . . for the evolving human spirit

HAMPTON ROADS PUBLISHING COMPANY publishes books
on a variety of subjects, including metaphysics, spiritu-
ality, health, visionary fiction, and other related topics.

For a copy of our latest trade catalog, call toll-free,
800-766-8009, or send your name and address to:

Hampton Roads Publishing Company, Inc.
1125 Stoney Ridge Road • Charlottesville, VA 22902
E-mail: hrpc@hrpub.com • Internet: www.hrpub.com